Staying Healthy Naturally

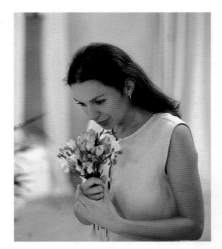

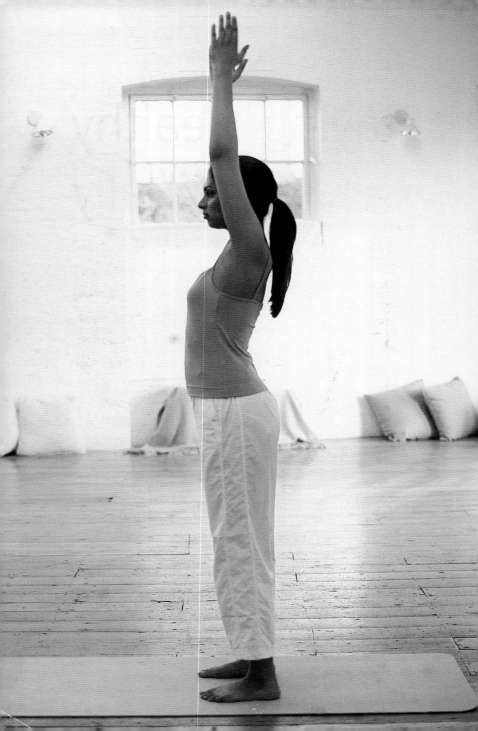

Staying Healthy
Naturally

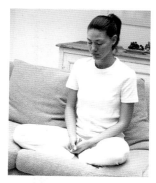

Over 250 practical techniques
and tips for health and
well-being including
aromatherapy, yoga,
meditation, nutrition,
massage and exercise

Tracey Kelly

southwater

2204 244 Bed 3/05

This edition is published by Southwater

Southwater is an imprint of
Anness Publishing Ltd
Hermes House, 88–89 Blackfriars Road
London SE1 8HA
tel. 020 7401 2077; fax 020 7633 9499
info@anness.com

© Anness Publishing Ltd 2005

UK agent: The Manning Partnership Ltd
6 The Old Dairy, Melcombe Road
Bath BA2 3LR
tel. 01225 478444; fax 01225 478440
sales@manning-partnership.co.uk

UK distributor: Grantham Book Services Ltd
Isaac Newton Way, Alma Park Industrial Estate
Grantham, Lincs NG31 9SD
tel. 01476 541080; fax 01476 541061
orders@gbs.tbs-ltd.co.uk

North American agent/distributor:
National Book Network
4501 Forbes Boulevard, Suite 200,
Lanham, MD 20706
tel. 301 459 3366; fax 301 429 5746
www.nbnbooks.com

Australian agent/distributor:
Pan Macmillan Australia
Level 18, St Martins Tower, 31 Market St,
Sydney, NSW 2000
tel. 1300 135 113; fax 1300 135 103
customer.service@macmillan.com.au

New Zealand agent/distributor:
David Bateman Ltd, 30 Tarndale Grove
Off Bush Road, Albany, Auckland
tel. (09) 415 7664; fax (09) 415 8892

A CIP catalogue record for this book is
available from the British Library.

Publisher: Joanna Lorenz
Editorial Director: Helen Sudell
Executive Editor: Joanne Rippin
Project Editor: Melanie Halton
Designer: Adele Morris, Jester Designs,
    Carlton Hibbert
Photographers: Sue Atkinson, Steve Baxter,
    Simon Bottomley, Martin Brigdale, Nick Cole,
    Nicky Dowey, James Duncan, Gus Filgate,
    John Freeman, Ian Garlick, Michelle Garrett,
    Christine Hanscomb, Amanda Heywood,
    Janine Hosegood, Alistair Hughes,
    Andrea Jones, Dave Jordan, Dave King,
    Don Last, William Lingwood, Lucy Mason,
    Liz McAuley, Steve Moss, Thomas Odulate,
    Lizzie Orme, Debbie Patterson,
    Anthony Pickhaver, Fiona Pragoff,
    Craig Robertson, Carin Simon, Simon Smith,
    Sam Stowell.
Production Controller: Claire Rae
Editorial Reader: Lindsay Zamponi

Previously published in five separate volumes,
50 Natural Ways to Energize, by Tracey Kelly
50 Natural Ways to Detox, by Tracey Kelly
50 Natural Ways to Stay Young, by Tracey Kelly
50 Natural Ways to Feel Sexy, by Jessica Dolland
50 Natural Ways to Sleep, by Tracey Kelly

10 9 8 7 6 5 4 3 2 1

Publisher's note:
The reader should not regard the
recommendations, ideas and techniques
expressed and described in this book as
substitutes for the advice of a qualified medical
practitioner or other qualified professional. Any
use to which the recommendations, ideas and
techniques are put is at the reader's sole
discretion and risk.

contents

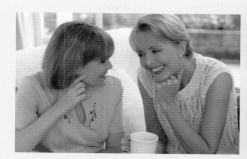

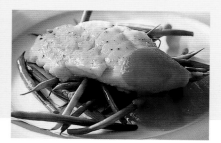

contents

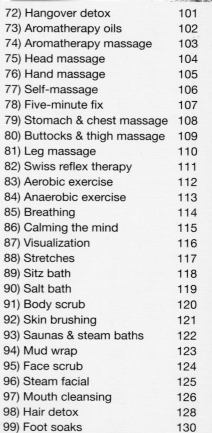

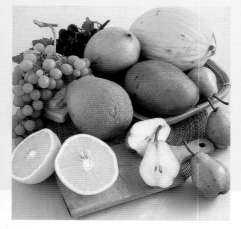

contents

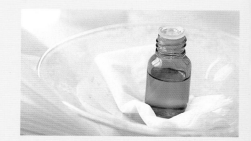

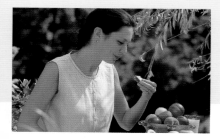

contents

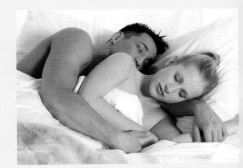

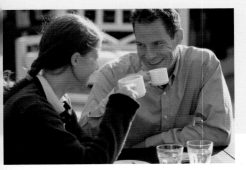

contents

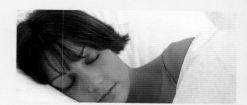
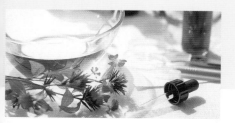

introduction

Our modern way of living has many benefits that make our lives much longer and potentially more enjoyable than ever before. But it has also become faster and busier, with many more demands on our time and personal resources. If we are not careful we can all too easily feel overwhelmed as the different strands of our existence – family, career, friends, study, health and leisure – compete for our attention. We may start to feel incapable, irritable, exhausted, depressed or permanently under the weather. At times like these, it pays to take stock of what is happening to us and to work out what we really want and need from life.

Fortunately, taking firm steps towards improving the overall quality of your life is easy, but you need to understand what is causing your difficulties so that you can address them. *Staying Healthy Naturally* has a holistic approach to improving your general well-being, emphasizing how nutrition, exercise, relaxation and rest, as well as rewarding relationships, are all crucial to a healthy lifestyle. This wealth of information is spread over five informative chapters.

In *Energize*, you will find out how you can turn your life around, replacing sluggishness and lethargy with boundless energy to meet the varied demands and challenges of each new day. It can be a matter of simply combining a nourishing diet with a rejuvenating exercise regime, but why not also try some powerful alternative therapies and indulge in invigorating pampering and relaxation techniques.

Detoxify is designed to help your body make a fresh start on the road to a healthier lifestyle. Flush out your system using a combination of detoxification diets and exercise, then complete the cleansing process using techniques for relaxing the mind and muscles, and finish off with a

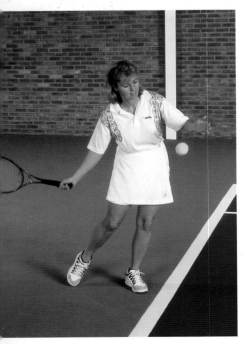

▲ *Energetic activity makes the heart and lungs stronger, and increases stamina.*

luxurious spa treatment. Once you've detoxed, you'll feel like you never want to eat junk food again.

Our increasing lifespan means that it is ever more important to discover ways of prolonging our health, improving our quality of life and "staying younger for longer". Making sure you care for yourself – body and soul – as you progress through life makes good sense, and in *Eternal Youth*, you'll discover just how you can do it.

Sex is an essential part of our lives, but unless we feel good about ourselves we can't feel sexy. *Feeling Sexy* is full of suggestions for improving your positive self-image, lifting your spirits and generally increasing your zest for life. As well as highlighting the importance of avoiding sexual "dampers" – stress, depression, tiredness, smoking, heavy drinking and even caffeine – it stresses the importance of sensitivity, communication, confidence and a good sense of humour. You will also discover how to involve every one of your senses for satisfying lovemaking.

A good night's sleep is essential for maintaining mental and physical health, and we soon suffer if this restorative process is regularly disrupted. In *Feel Sleepy*, there are lots of tips for ensuring a peaceful night's sleep. Relaxing exercises and pampering treatments will help you wind down at the end of a stressful

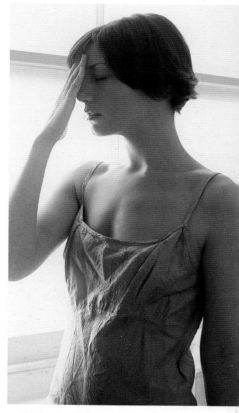

▲ *Taking stock of your situation can help you to focus on your priorities.*

day, and there are suggestions for making your sleeping environment more relaxing. If your sleep pattern is out of your control, there is advice on how you can go about improving the situation. You will also learn about the function of dreams and how you can control and enjoy them.

With all this helpful information, you can take control of every aspect of your life and learn to enjoy it to the full.

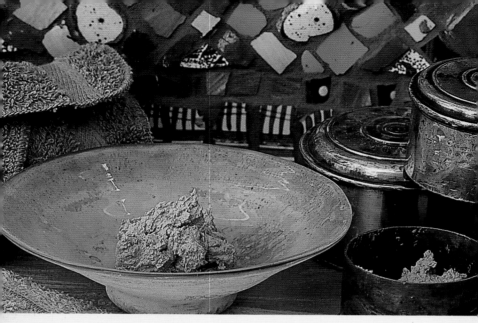

energize

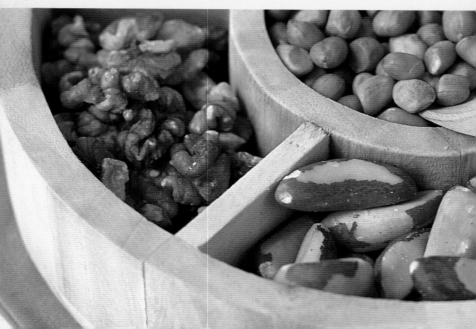

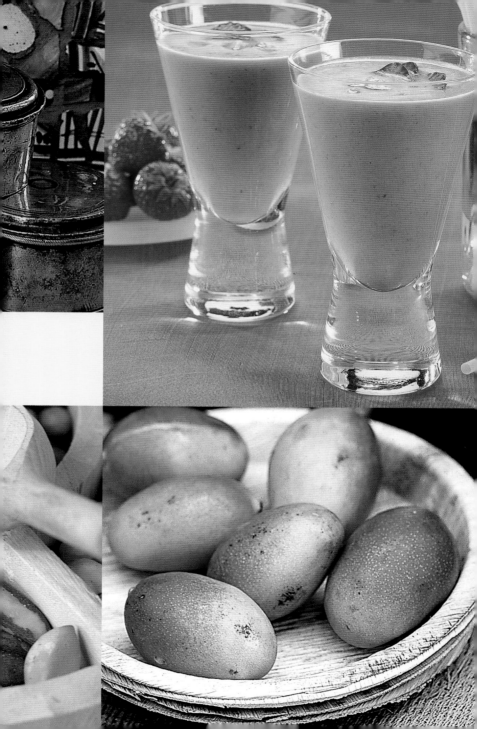

▾ *Making your health your number one priority will provide you with energy for a full and happy life.*

learn to energize

As the pace of life in the 21st century becomes ever faster, some of us are left wondering, "Where will I ever find the energy to do all the things I need to do? Will I ever have some time left over for myself?"

The demands of partners, family, career, study, health and leisure pursuits seem to scream for constant attention. Whenever you are feeling frazzled and exhausted, bear in mind that you cannot do everything, and you can choose those people and things that are important to you. By making sure that you take care of yourself, you will ensure that you have the energy levels to deal with situations, happily and effectively.

This chapter sets out to help you uncover the great reserves of energy available to you, both physical and mental. By learning to pace yourself, you can accomplish all of your tasks — and still find time for yourself.

taking stock

It can be a real revelation to take a day off to sort out your priorities: this alone will have a restorative effect on your vitality. The mind can easily go into overdrive, leaving you going around in circles and achieving nothing productive; taking steps to review your current expenditure of energy can help you "spend" it in more positive, efficient ways.

Maybe you've been grabbing junk food on the go, and perhaps you just haven't found the time to go swimming or play that game of squash in weeks. Could your insomnia be due to the huge amount of caffeine you've consumed to get you through the day? Maybe you've been feeling overwhelmed by the apparent seriousness of your life and its lack of enjoyment and fun.

You have a vague notion that your sluggish, lethargic feelings may be connected to these points, but you are unsure of what steps to take to correct the imbalances that harmful stimulants may have caused in the past.

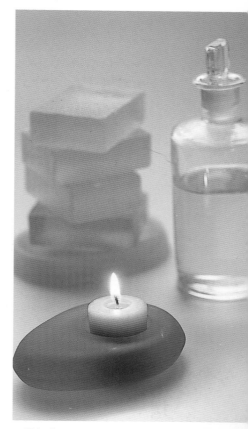

▲ Take time out to pamper yourself with invigorating bath oils and fragrances.

energizing nutrition

It has often been said that "you are what you eat", and recent medical research has proved the validity of this old adage. Keeping a close watch on your daily diet – eating from a variety of fresh, unprocessed organic foods; staying hydrated by drinking plenty of water and low-caffeine herbal teas; keeping alcohol consumption at a moderate level – will ensure that you stay fit and alert. In particular, choosing foods that provide a good supply of the antioxidants – vitamins A, C and E – will help protect you from harmful pollution and chemicals in the environment, and waylay the onset of degenerative diseases.

rejuvenating exercise

Many people are surprised when they discover that physical activity actually gives them more energy, not less. Exercise oxygenates the bloodstream and boosts the metabolism, providing a lasting stream of energy. And the long-term benefits of regular exercise are well-documented: it tones the muscles and works the heart, giving you a fighting chance for a fitter body as you grow older. By releasing substances called endorphins, it also helps to elevate your mood, leaving you in a brighter, more positive frame of mind that prepares you to face daily challenges with greater ease.

For maximum health value, it is best to include both aerobic and anaerobic exercises. Aerobic exercises are those that raise the pulse, burn fat, boost the immune system and exercise the heart, helping to prevent the build-up of arterial deposits that can lead to heart disease, one of the major killers. Walking, swimming, tennis, cycling and ball games provide a good workout and are enjoyable.

Anaerobics strengthen and tone the muscles, and build bone density, keeping at bay degenerative illnesses such as osteoporosis and back and joint problems. Examples include exercises where the muscles work at high intensity for short periods of time, such as weight lifting, squash and circuit training.

powerful therapies
The healing powers of alternative therapies provide ways to work through physical and mental problems, and many are meditative and relaxing. Their effectiveness increases with regular use. Tactile therapies such as massage and reflexology work by manipulating muscles and pressure points to ease

pain and discomfort. Colour and crystal healing use the energies of subtle vibrations to enliven and protect. With aromatherapy, the potent, active essences of plants and herbs are inhaled or absorbed through the skin – and their scent alone provides a delightful mood lift.

sensual pampering
It is important not to forget that feeling attractive is an essential part of your energizing plan. Pampering your body with the delicious fragrances and textures of some of the spa treatments included in this chapter will help you to look and feel your best. Invigorating body scrubs and bath oils cleanse and hydrate the skin, and homemade hair rinses and skin fresheners prepare you to face the world with renewed grace and beauty.

lighten your load
Contrary to popular belief, taking regular breaks from normal activity actually increases your productivity, whether at work, at home or in dealing with family matters. Especially when under stress, taking time out to "recharge the batteries" can be a life-saver. It is easy to carry out self-help practices, from deep breathing techniques to taking a walk around the block – often, it is simply a matter of remembering to do so. Enjoyable activities such as dancing and having a laugh enliven your spirits, giving you the motivation to perform all the practical tasks you have to accomplish.

▼ *A diet that includes a variety of fresh, nutritious foods is the best recipe for staying vibrant and active.*

energizing treatments

Increase your vitality by choosing from the following ideas for fighting fatigue and giving yourself an energizing boost, whether short or longer term. A selection of revitalizing foods, drinks, vitamins, exercises, beauty treatments and therapies will help set you on the road to a fit and healthy body and a lively, productive mind.

Diet is an important part of an active lifestyle, and it is essential that you get enough nutrients from food. Here you will find information on the health-giving properties of meat, fish and poultry; fruits and vegetables; grains, nuts and pulses. You'll also find recipes for delicious juices, tisanes and shakes.

Aerobic, t'ai chi and yoga exercises are all satisfying ways to increase your physical stamina. Also included are reflexology, aromatherapy and crystal healing therapies, which improve the body's flow of energy. Instant energy fixes such as clearing your mind will remind you that you have the power to make your life as fulfilling and exciting as it can be.

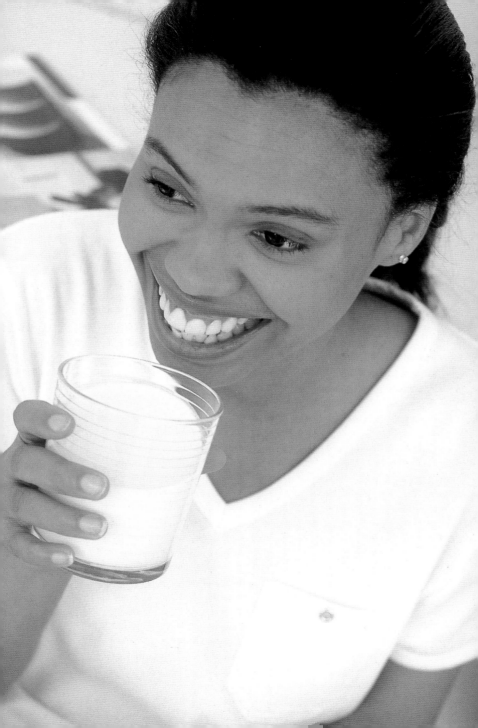

1 vital vitamin C

This important energizing vitamin is essential for maintaining a healthy and resilient immune system. Vitamin C helps the body absorb iron from vegetable sources. It also helps fight off colds and flu.

Also known as ascorbic acid, vitamin C assists with tissue growth, the healing of wounds, and the prevention of blood clotting and bruising. It is a powerful antioxidant, which – when taken with vitamins A and E – helps curtail the effects of pollution on the body. A shortage of vitamin C can result in water retention, a lack of energy, poor digestion, colds and bronchial infections. Some good food sources of vitamin C include berries, citrus fruits, green leafy vegetables, guavas, tomatoes, melons and peppers.

cooking care

Vitamin C is particularly unstable and is easily destroyed by heat, so it is a good idea to get your intake by eating plenty of fresh, raw fruits and vegetables. It is best to buy organic produce, and prepare just before eating to preserve as much of the vitamin content as possible. Keep a well-stocked fruit bowl for a quick energy boost between meals.

▸ *Oranges and lemons provide the body with a very accessible form of vitamin C.*

SUPPLEMENTS
As a supplement, vitamin C is more effective if it is taken along with bioflavonoids, calcium and magnesium (it aids calcium absorption). The RDA is only 60mg, but many health practitioners recommend higher doses to keep disease at bay – somewhere between 200-500mg for healthy adults. If you feel you need more vitamin C, consult your doctor before taking larger amounts.

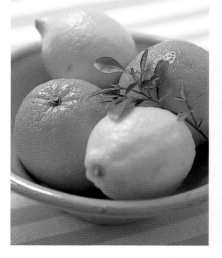

2   rejuvenating vitamin E

An essential fat-soluble substance, vitamin E helps increase stamina and endurance and, not only does it promote fertility, it is reported to spice up your sex life as well.

Vitamin E contains several antioxidant compounds that help the body fight free radicals, to which we all are vulnerable via pollution and food additives. Vitamin E is also known to prevent degenerative diseases such as heart disease, arthritis, diabetes and cancer. Plenty of vitamin E keeps your skin looking younger and glowing, and actually helps keep wrinkles at bay. Vitamin E oil can be used on the skin as a soothing, topical treatment for eczema, cold sores, skin ulcers and shingles. A deficiency in vitamin E is not very common, but signs may include fatigue, premature aging, inflamed varicose or thread veins, and wounds that are slow to heal.

how to get it

Vitamin E is found in many types of foods, including nuts, seeds such as sunflower and pumpkin, cold-pressed oils, vegetables, spinach, whole grains, wheatgerm oil, asparagus, avocado, beef, seafood, apples, carrots and celery. As a food supplement, vitamin E is best taken with other antioxidants – vitamin C, betacarotene (vitamin A) and selenium; an element important in maintaining a healthy immune system and enhancing a positive frame of mind. The RDA for women is 8mg and around 10mg for men.

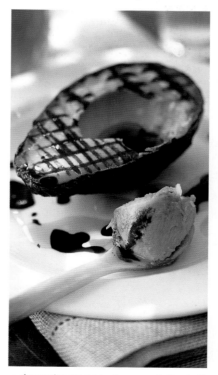

▲ *Avocados are a good source of vitamin E. Eat them as a starter or as part of a salad.*

B-complex vitamins

The B group vitamins are vital for their role in releasing energy from food, providing the body with a steady stream of nutrients. Eat a variety of B-rich foods, as they work in tandem with each other.

The best way to get B vitamins is from natural food sources, although there are many good-quality B-complex supplements available. Vegetarians in particular may need to top up their B_{12} intake by using a supplement. Care should be taken, as a sensitivity to niacin may result in a temporary rash or headache for 15–30 minutes. The B vitamins are better taken in the early part of the day, as they provide a real physical and mental boost.

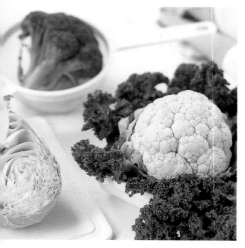

▲ Like vitamin C, Bs are water soluble and easily destroyed – take care when cooking.

CRUCIAL B VITAMINS

• Vitamin B_1 (thiamin): Enhances circulation; boosts brain power. Foods: seeds, beans, peanuts, bran, liver, pork, seafood, egg-yolk.

• Vitamin B_2 (riboflavin): Helps metabolize amino acids, fatty acids and carbohydrates. Foods: nuts, eggs, dairy, vegetables, meats.

• Vitamin B_3 (niacin): Promotes circulation, healthy skin and nerves. Foods: liver, poultry, fish, rabbit, nuts, yeast, cereals, legumes.

• Vitamin B_5 (pantothenic acid): Aids hormone secretion; helps fight allergies. Foods: beef, eggs, fish, kidney, legumes, mushrooms.

• Vitamin B_6 (pyridoxine): Helps balance female hormones and fight depression. Foods: chicken, fish, liver, kidney, eggs, walnuts, carrots.

• Vitamin B_9: Aids red blood cell formation. Foods: spinach, beans, broccoli, vegetables, whole grains.

• Vitamin B_{12} (cyanocobamin): Helps sharpen mental processes. Foods: liver, red meat, shellfish, eggs, cheese, fish.

4 essential minerals

Energizing minerals such as magnesium, zinc and iron play a vital role in regulating the body's functions. They are constituents of all body tissues and fluids, and work to stimulate the immune system.

invigorating magnesium

Take plenty of magnesium to boost energy levels – a deficiency can lead to tiredness and irritability. It helps the body absorb calcium, so it is important for the formation of bone and teeth, and also helps control blood pressure. To consume enough of the mineral, choose from a wide selection of magnesium-rich foods, including dairy products, fish, meat, legumes, apples, apricots, avocados, bananas, wholegrain cereals, nuts, dark green vegetables and cocoa.

activating zinc

Especially important for the growth of muscle tissue and for maintaining a healthy and active immune system, zinc is often used with vitamin C to fight colds, sore throats and flu. Skin problems such as acne also benefit

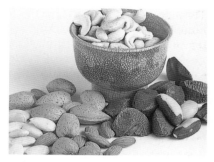

▲ Nuts are bursting with essential minerals such as zinc, magnesium and selenium.

from zinc, and a good supply will keep hair, skin and nails healthy. To get enough zinc, eat plenty of meat, poultry, fish, nuts, eggs, seeds, whole grains and brewer's yeast.

energizing iron

Essential in the production of red blood cells, iron is important for sustaining energy levels. Symptoms of deficiency include fatigue, muscular weakness, nervousness and shortness of breath. Include liver, meat, egg yolks, dark green leafy vegetables, legumes and nuts in your diet. Orange juice drunk with a vegetarian meal will help the body absorb iron.

> **CAUTION**
> Before taking any type of iron supplement, consult your doctor, as iron can be harmful in large doses. A fatal dose for children could be as little as 600mg.

5 vitalizing fruit & vegetables

Fruit and vegetables are storehouses of energizing nutrients. Packed with vitamins, minerals, fibre and enzymes, raw fruit and vegetables are the perfect snack, and are easy to eat at any time of day.

refreshing fruit

Fruit such as apples, pears, mangoes, strawberries and grapes provide a steady stream of energy via fructose, a natural sugar. Apples also contain malic acid, which boosts digestion. Citrus fruits are packed with vitamin C, a powerful antioxidant that protects the body against harmful free radicals, inhibits premature aging and increases iron absorption. Freshly squeezed oranges and grapefruits stimulate the digestion and tone the whole system. They are also a good source of betacarotene, calcium, phosphorus and potassium.

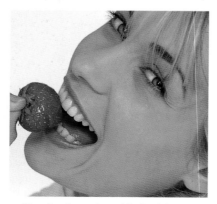

▲ *Strawberries make an ideal quick snack.*

handy dried fruit

Higher in calories than fresh fruit, dried fruit provides plenty of sustaining energy for a busy day. Unlike other high-sugar foods, such as chocolate and sweets, dried fruit is an excellent source of nutrients. For an easily portable, fast energy snack, look for unsulphured fruit, such as dried hunza apricots, figs, dates, raisins, currants, apples and peaches.

vitamin-rich vegetables

Known for their calming effect on the body, vegetables balance acid and alkaline levels and provide essential nutrients. A large salad at lunchtime will fill you up and is satisfyingly crunchy. Raw spinach is an excellent choice – it contains betacarotene (vitamin A), vitamin C, calcium, folate, iron, potassium, thiamin and zinc.

With a rich supply of vitamin A, carrots have the effect of stimulating the whole body. They are easy to clean and carry for a quick snack. Members of the cruciferous family – broccoli, cauliflower, cabbage, Brussels sprouts and watercress – stimulate the liver, and keep the digestive system active.

grilled mango with lime syrup and sorbet

If you want to serve this dessert as part of a larger barbecue meal, cook the mangoes in advance using a griddle set over the first red-hot coals, then set them aside until you are ready.

250g/9oz/1¼ cups sugar
juice of 6 limes
3 star anise
6 small or 3 medium to large mangoes
groundnut (peanut) oil, for brushing

Place the sugar in a heavy pan and add 250ml/8fl oz/1 cup water. Heat gently until the sugar has dissolved. Increase the heat and boil for 5 minutes. Cool completely. Add the lime juice and any pulp left in the squeezer. Strain the mixture and reserve 200m/7fl oz/scant 1 cup in a bowl with the star anise.

Pour the remaining liquid into a measuring jug or cup and make up to 600ml/1 pint/2½ cups with cold water. Mix well and pour into a freezerproof container. Freeze for 1½ hours, stir well and return to the freezer for another hour until set.

Transfer the sorbet mixture to a processor and pulse to a smooth icy purée. Freeze for another hour or longer, if wished. Alternatively, make the sorbet in an ice-cream maker; it

will take about 20 minutes, and should then be frozen for at least 30 minutes before serving.

Pour the reserved syrup into a pan and boil for 2–3 minutes, or until thickened a little. Leave to cool. Cut the cheeks from either side of the stone on each unpeeled mango, and score the flesh on each in a diamond pattern. Brush with a little oil. Heat a griddle until very hot and a few drops of water sprinkled on the surface evaporate instantly. Lower the heat a little and grill the mango halves, cut-side down, for 30–60 seconds until branded with golden grill marks.

Invert the mango cheeks on individual plates and serve hot or cold with the syrup drizzled over and a scoop or two of sorbet. Decorate with the reserved star anise.

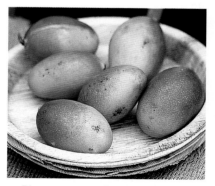

▲ *Ripe mangoes are heady with flavour. Eat them on their own or made into a dessert.*

6 healthy whole grains

Whole grains and cereals are vital ingredients in a healthy, energizing diet. Not only are they an excellent source of low-fat protein, they contain carbohydrates, fibre, vitamins and minerals.

bountiful grains

Humans have been eating grains for millennia, and these wholesome foods were probably among the first agricultural crops. Western diets tend to rely more on refined cereals than whole grains, but this is at the cost of valuable nutrients and essential fibre.

Wholegrain cereals are an excellent source of vegetable protein, iron, energy-releasing B vitamins and vitamin E. They contain complex, unrefined carbohydrates, which, because they are digested more slowly than other nutrients, release a steady stream of sugar into the blood.

To glean a variety of the best nutrients, include a selection of different grains in your diet, such as brown rice, barley, millet, oats, buckwheat and quinoa, and eat them at different times of the day.

For a breakfast with staying power, try a bowl of porridge – oats absorb impurities in the blood, leaving your skin glowing. For lunch or supper, a bowl of brown rice with lightly steamed vegetables will work to steady the nervous system. For tasty variety, you can add a few chopped nuts, raisins

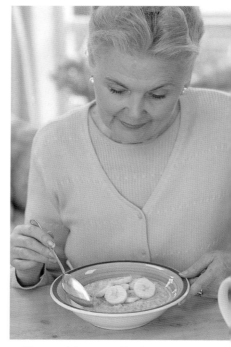

▲ The starch in oat porridge helps to keep blood sugar levels on an even keel.

or apricots. Quinoa, the South American grain, contains more protein than any other, and so is a good choice for times when you need to be on top form all day long.

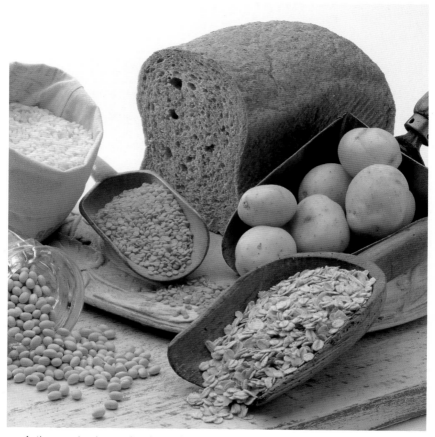

▲ *Active people who require plenty of stamina should eat wholegrain cereals, because they release a steady stream of energy into the blood and are digested slowly.*

essential fibre

Unprocessed whole grains are a good source of dietary fibre, both soluble and insoluble, and contain much more than refined cereals do. Fibre is crucial for the prevention of constipation and serious, life-threatening diseases such as colon and rectal cancers, ulcers and heart disease. Fibre also binds with harmful cholesterol and so helps it to be eliminated from the body.

Wholegrain bread is a good source of fibre; aim to eat about six slices a day, without butter. Vary the types so that you include different grains, for example, alternating wholewheat, rye, multigrain, oat and millet. For additional variety, look out for the many wholegrain versions of international breads, such as naan bread and chapatis, or Scandinavian and German rye breads.

7

energy-sustaining pulses

Providing essential low-fat protein, fibre and vitamins, pulses have long been a staple of vegetarian diets. They are bursting with minerals – including folate, iron, magnesium and potassium.

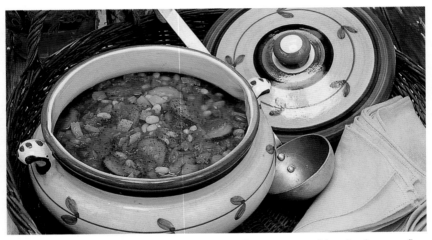

large choice

Pulses include beans and legumes such as lentils, dried peas, pinto and mung beans, chickpeas and soya beans. It is preferable to use dry beans in cooking, as processing often adds sugar and salt. For a nourishing and energy-giving lunch, try eating a stew or thick soup made from a selection of tasty beans and vegetables. Alternatively, try delicious baked dishes based on butter (lima) or pinto beans.

Most dried beans need to be soaked for at least eight hours before cooking. Leave overnight in a covered

▲ *Bean soups provide a steady energy flow through the slow release of carbohydrates.*

pan with plenty of cold water. The next morning, drain and rinse before boiling hard for at least 10 minutes, then leave them to simmer until cooked. Alternatively, follow your recipe for cooking instructions.

bean sensitivity

Never eat beans raw or partially cooked; they may cause an allergic reaction. When trying a new type of bean, eat a small amount first to test.

8 brain-boosting fish

Fish is often called "brain food" as it is high in protein, B vitamins, minerals and Omega fatty acids. It is best to include several varieties as part of your energizing diet.

White fish is a good choice as it is very low in fat. Oily fish – such as sardines, mackerel, herring, tuna, trout and salmon – provide large amounts of vitamins A and D. They also provide Omega fatty acids, which are beneficial in helping to prevent coronary heart diseases, and leave the skin looking fresh and clear.

choice cooking methods
There are a number of fast and delicious ways to cook fish. Almost any cooking method suits fish except boiling, although simmering is fine for healthy soups.

Since fish is so delicate, it is better to undercook than overcook it. Because of many factors – the variety, weight and thickness of the flesh – it is impossible to give exact cooking times for a portion of fish, but it is considered cooked when the internal temperature has reached 63^0C/145^0F.

Fish can be baked, braised, fried, stir-fried, grilled (broiled), barbecued, microwaved and seared. To test whether fish fillets are done, part the flesh with a small knife; the flesh should look opaque rather than translucent. Next, gently ease the flesh off the bone; it should come away but not fall off easily.

cold preparation
Very fresh fish may be prepared without heat by being marinated or soused with lemon juice or flavoured vinegar – the acids soften the flesh and turn it opaque. One classic dish that uses this method is ceviche, where cubes or strips of firm white fish, such as halibut, cod, snapper and turbot, are marinated in lemon juice, salt and chopped chillis for two hours. Japanese sushi uses very fresh fish often rolled in seaweed, and garnished with vinegar and wasabi, a very hot mustard.

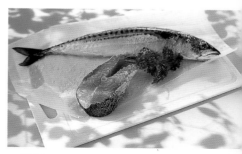

▲ Fish is an ideal food – it is a delicious source of protein and important nutrients.

9 wholesome eggs

Eggs contain the most complete nutrition of any food – all encased in a tidy package with a long shelf-life. They provide energy-boosting protein, iron, zinc and vitamins A, E and B complex.

a good egg

Easily accessible and inexpensive, eggs can be a wonderful addition to a healthy and energizing diet. When eaten in moderation, there is no need to fear excessive intake of cholesterol. Made up of white (albumen) and yolk, an egg consists of water, fat and protein, with smaller amounts of other essential nutrients and minerals. The white contains water and protein, while the yolk contains fat, protein and vitamins. To take advantage of their complete nutrition, eggs should be enjoyed whole; organic, free-range (farm-fresh) varieties of chicken and duck eggs offer the best quality and taste.

the perfect ingredient

Eggs are easy to cook and incredibly versatile, lending themselves to many exciting dishes such as omelettes, quiches, frittatas, custards and soufflés. They also provide a quick and delicious meal on their own, following one of many cooking methods: they can be hard- or soft-boiled, fried, scrambled, poached or baked.

Controlling the heat and cooking time are the keys to preparing eggs successfully. Generally, when making plain cooked eggs, the temperature should not be too high – they can easily burn, as in frying; or they may lose taste and texture when over-boiled, poached or baked.

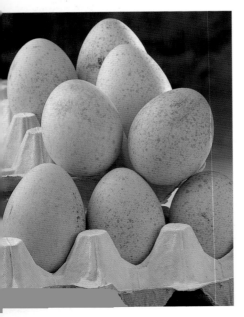

◄ *With so many egg dishes to choose from – both sweet and savoury – you're bound to find an energizing recipe to suit your tastes.*

10 protein-packed poultry

A good source of quality protein, B vitamins and some iron, poultry is also low in fat if the skin is removed. Preferably choose organic, free-range poultry to ensure it is healthy and nutritious.

light meal, anytime

Ideal for use in an energizing diet, high-protein chicken and other poultry such as turkey, duck and guinea fowl offer many benefits in terms of nutrition and taste. Poultry is extremely versatile and complements many side dishes: vegetables, potatoes, grains such as rice and couscous, and even fruit – it is delicious prepared with tangy apricots and cranberries.

preparing poultry

Poultry may be used whole or cut into pieces for cooking. It can be prepared using a variety of methods, from grilling (broiling), baking and frying, to barbecuing, roasting and boiling; or it can be added to a variety of casseroles, soups and stir-fries.

It is essential to arrive at the right cooking time and temperature: poultry must never be eaten undercooked, as bacteria may be lurking; and if overcooked, the meat will be tough and stringy.

To make roast chicken – one of the easiest and most delicious poultry dishes – use the following guidelines: preheat the oven to 200°C/400°F/Gas 6.

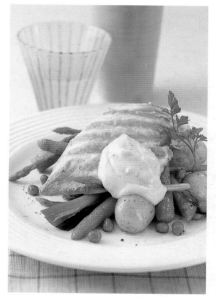

▲ Escalopes of chicken are quick and easy to prepare – they are simple, tasty and highly nutritious.

Weigh the bird after it has been trimmed and stuffed, and place in a roasting pan in the hot oven. Allow 20 minutes of cooking time per 450g/1lb, plus an extra 20 minutes. With a very large bird, cover with foil until the final 15 minutes of cooking.

11

iron-rich meat & game

Although the general health advice is to moderate your intake of red meat, thus reducing saturated fat, it is still the best source of readily absorbed iron, zinc and B vitamins – all crucial for boosting energy.

Today's meat is leaner than formerly, and if low-fat cooking methods are used, it can fit into the profile of a healthy diet and provide you with plenty of sustained energy. Choose organic lamb, beef and pork, and free-range game to ensure that the meat is safe, free from hormones and additives, and comes from farms where animal welfare is a priority.

Pan frying is probably the most traditional way of cooking beef or game sirloins, fillets and chops. Start by taking a heavy pan, preferably non-stick, and rub it with just a light coating of sunflower or safflower oil. Heat the pan and add a knob (pat) of butter, which should melt immediately.

Trim excess fat from the steak or chop, and cook following the times given below. Use a draining spoon or fish slice (metal spatula) to transfer the steak to the plate. You can then serve with a selection of side dishes, such as rice or potatoes, roasted or stir-fried vegetables and green salads.

cooking times for red meat

For very rare steak: cut about 2.5cm/1in thick and allow 1 minute for each side for fillet; for rump (round steak), allow 2 minutes per side.

For rare steak: allow 2 minutes each side for fillet; 3 minutes for rump.

For medium rare steak: allow 2–3 minutes for each side for fillet; 2–4 minutes for rump.

For well-done steak: allow 3 minutes each side, then reduce heat and allow a further 5–10 minutes.

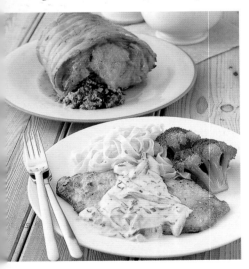

◀ *Include meat in your diet to supply your body with a full range of nutrients.*

12 essential fats & oils

Choosing the right fat is vital for sustaining energy levels and overall health. Plant oils provide essential fatty acids and vitamin E, beneficial for heart and skin. Animal fats should be used in moderation.

While butter and cream may be eaten occasionally, plant oils offer a healthier option for supplying essential energizing nutrients found in fats. High in unsaturated fats, olive, sunflower, safflower and grapeseed oils are all good choices to include in your daily diet. Speciality oils such as walnut, sesame, almond and hazelnut are a tasty alternative. Some of the essential substances in oils are lost during heated processing, so look for organic, cold-pressed oils, which retain most of their nutritional value.

mediterranean olive dressing
250ml/8fl oz/1 cup olive oil
120ml/4fl oz/½ cup freshly squeezed
    lemon juice
50ml/2fl oz/¼ cup water
10ml/2 tsps brown sugar
2.5ml/½ tsp each of oregano, thyme,
    sage and marjoram
salt and freshly ground black pepper

Place oil, lemon juice and water in a bottle. Add the herbs, then a dash of salt and black pepper. Shake well and add the dressing to salads or use as a marinade for roast vegetables.

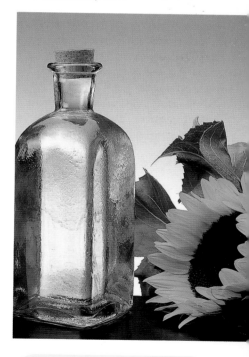

▼ The delicate flavour of sunflower oil will not overpower any dish.

REVITALIZING
Almond oil is an excellent choice for a revitalizing massage, as it is easily absorbed into the skin.

13

nutritious nuts & seeds

Protein-rich nuts and seeds give a more sustained energy boost than carbohydrates, and are a good alternative to meat. The vitamin E content of nuts also helps the condition of skin, hair and nails.

Nuts contain essential nutrients, such as B vitamins, calcium, iron, potassium, magnesium, phosphorus and essential fatty acids. They also contain selenium – just three brazil nuts provide the daily requirement.

versatile nuts

Walnuts, almonds, cashews, hazelnuts, brazil nuts and peanuts offer some of the best health benefits – they can be eaten on their own, or added to porridge, breads, casseroles and salads. Since they have a high oil content (albeit unsaturated), keep in mind that nuts are high in calories and should be eaten in moderation.

nutritious seeds

Seeds such as pumpkin, sunflower and sesame offer similar nutritional values with slightly fewer calories. Buy them in small quantities, seal and store in a cool place. Wholegrain toast spread with tahini (crushed sesame seed spread) or peanut butter makes a nutritious start to the day, and will provide energy all morning.

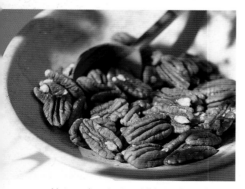

▲ Nuts make a tasty addition to cereals and porridge. You can also add them to stir-fries, breads, cakes and biscuits (cookies).

▶ For sustained energy, eat a handful of nuts before exercising, or take some along while outdoors on a long hike.

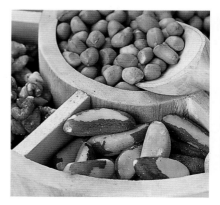

14 cleansing garlic

Containing antiviral and antibacterial nutrients, garlic acts to cleanse and energize the immune system. It is said to protect against disease and bacteria, lower cholesterol levels and fight cancer.

The plant's historical use has been documented for 5,000 years. Often called nature's strongest antibiotic, it was used to prevent the plague in France in the early 1700s, and in the trenches to fight gangrene in World Wars I and II. Garlic is reputed to bestow all kinds of health benefits, from increasing overall physical strength and vitality, to reducing lethargy – so if you're feeling "under the weather" generally, a good place to start energizing may be to up your intake of garlic.

tasty addition
Add fresh garlic to olive or walnut oil for a piquant salad dressing. It is also delicious cooked in main dishes such as stir-fries, casseroles and soups. If you do not like the taste or smell of garlic, try taking deodorized garlic supplements, which are available from health food shops and chemists.

garlic bread
Another delicious way to boost your intake is to make garlic bread as part of a lunch or dinner menu. Crush two bulbs of garlic and infuse in

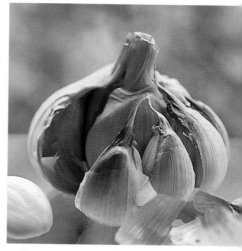

▲ Garlic is one of the most renowned "miracle cures" in nearly all cultures. It is added to many dishes – even desserts!

120ml/4 fl oz/½ cup of olive oil an hour previous to serving time. Take slices of wholemeal (whole-wheat), rye, mixed grain or white bread, and brush each side with the garlic oil. Heat until slightly crisp in a preheated oven (160°C/325°F/Gas 3) for 10-15 minutes, depending on the thickness of the slices. Serve warm with pasta or a ragout of vegetables.

15 healthy hydration

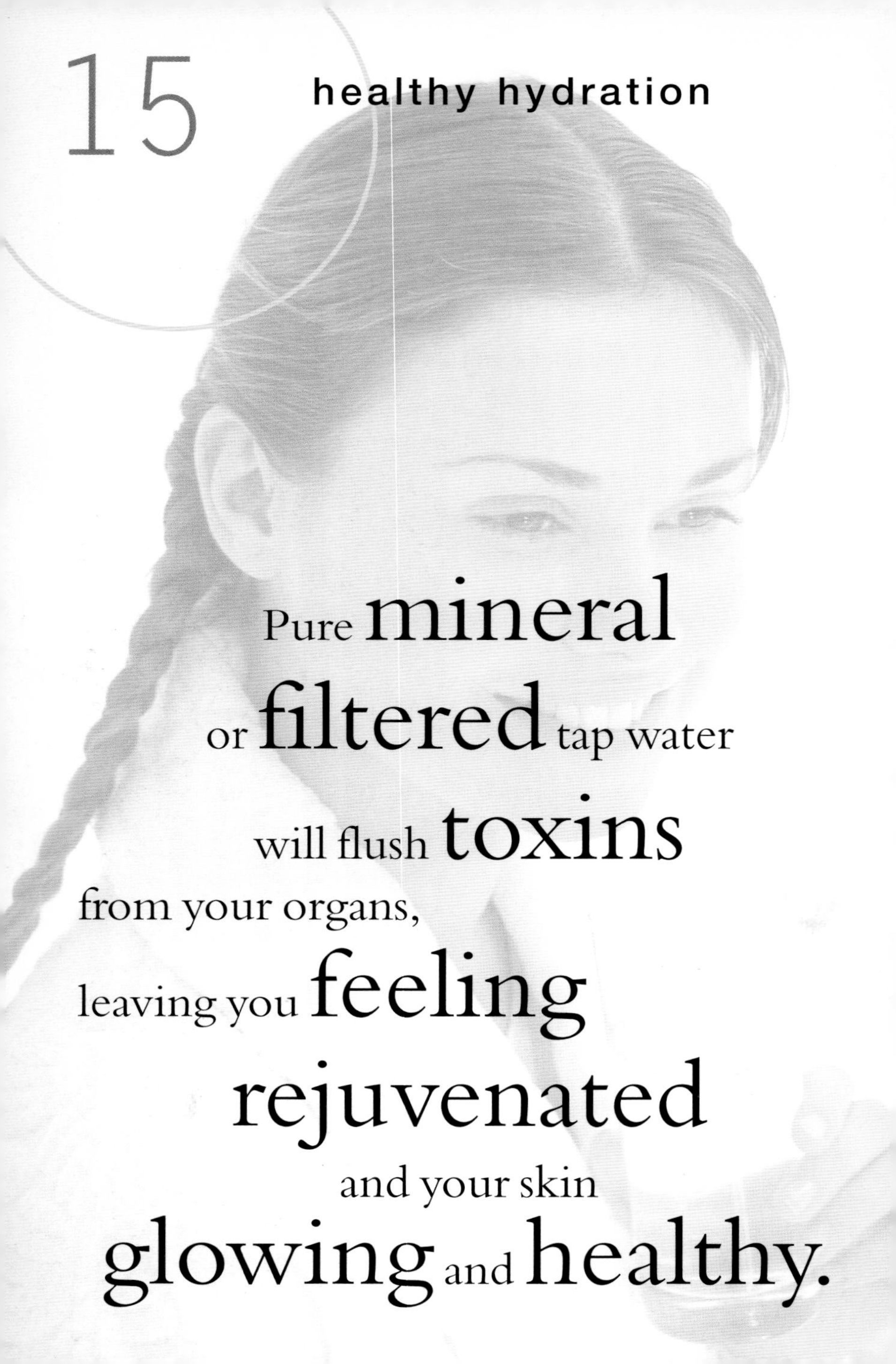

Pure **mineral** or **filtered** tap water will flush **toxins** from your organs, leaving you **feeling rejuvenated** and your skin **glowing** and **healthy.**

16 fruit & vegetable juices

Fresh fruit and vegetable juices are an ideal way to give yourself an energy boost. They stimulate the system, providing fructose – a slow-burning sugar – and plentiful vitamins and minerals.

cranberry and apple juice
This refreshing juice boosts the metabolism first thing in the morning.

4 eating apples
600ml/1 pint/2½ cups cranberry juice
2.5cm/1 in fresh root ginger,
    peeled and grated

Peel the apples, if you wish, then core and chop them. Pour the cranberry juice into the food processor or blender, then add the apples and ginger and process for a few minutes until smooth. Serve chilled.

zingy vegetable juice
The ginger in this juice packs a powerful punch, giving you a lift in the afternoon.

1 beetroot (beet), cooked in its
    natural juice
1 large carrot, sliced
4cm/1½ in piece fresh root ginger,
    peeled and grated
2 apples, peeled, cored and chopped
150g/5oz/1¼ cups seedless
    white grapes
300ml/½ pints fresh orange juice

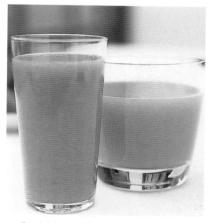

▲ Fresh blended juices are easy to make.

Place the beetroot, carrot, ginger, apples, grapes and orange juice in a food processor or blender and process for a few minutes until smooth. Serve immediately, or chill and serve later.

JUICING TIPS
• Juices speed up the metabolism and improve energy levels.
• Drink fruit juices with breakfast – their sugars kick-start the system.
• Vegetable juices are best drunk in the afternoon, as they re-establish the body's acid and alkaline balance.

Herbal teas
hydrate and refresh
the body
without straining the
cardio-vascular system.
Mint tea is especially
stimulating when
energy levels are low.

18 fragrant tisanes

Tisanes are teas made by seeping sprigs of garden-fresh leaves and flowers in boiling water. They provide a treat for the senses, and can give you an instant physical and psychological boost.

The experience of drinking tisanes is a little bit like taking the garden's growing energy into your body. The wonderful fragrances of these clean and clear tonics act as mood enhancers, and they provide a visual treat – as well as tasting wonderfully fresh. Many blossoms can be used for making tisanes, such as dandelion, rosemary, rose petals, lavender, lime blossom, peppermint, lemon verbena, jasmine and bergamot.

rosemary tisane

This familiar garden plant contains several active, aromatic oils. The action of rosemary is such that it stimulates as it increases the blood supply to the brain, keeping the mind clear and aiding concentration. Rosemary will also relieve nervous tension and combat fatigue. It is ideal from a culinary point of view, in that it is a sturdy evergreen shrub, from which leaf sprigs can be cut all year round.

To make a tea, place one sprig of rosemary (or 10ml/2 tsp dried herb) in a cup and add 250ml/8fl oz/ 1 cup boiling water. Infuse for 4 minutes before removing the sprig.

▾ *A wonderful way to revive tired senses, tisanes are tasty and aromatic.*

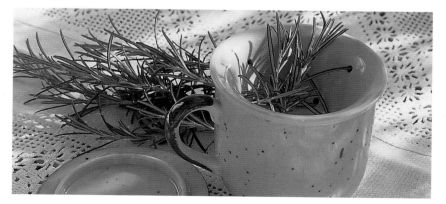

19 fruit shakes

More nutritious than the fat- and calorie-laden ice-cream variety, fresh fruit shakes supply an immediate and lasting burst of fructose, providing you with sustained energy for hours.

mixed berry yogurt shake

250ml/8fl oz/1 cup semi-skimmed milk, chilled
250ml/8fl oz/1 cup low-fat natural yogurt
115g/4oz mixed berries
5ml/1 tsp rosewater
a little honey, to taste

Blend the milk, yogurt, fruits and rosewater in a food processor, and process until frothy. Add honey to taste; this will depend on the sweetness of the fruits. Pour into tall glasses and serve.

citrus shake

1 pineapple
6 oranges, peeled and chopped
1 lemon, juiced
1 pink grapefruit, peeled and chopped

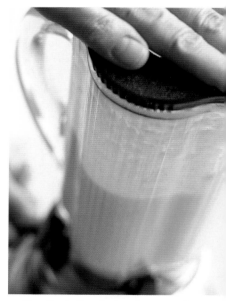

▲ The vitamin C and mineral content of fruit shakes provides much of the RDA – and they are wonderfully tasty, too!

Prepare the pineapple by cutting the bottom and spiky top off the fruit. Stand upright and cut off the skin, removing all the spikes and as little of the flesh as possible.

Lay the pineapple on its side and cut into bite-size chunks. Place the pineapple, oranges, lemon juice and grapefruit in a food processor or blender, and process for a few minutes until the ingredients are combined. Press the fruit juice through a sieve to remove any pith or membranes. Serve chilled with breakfast or a snack.

20 fruit smoothies

A combination of soft-textured fruits and yogurt, smoothies are easy to make and offer a tasty alternative to eating plain fruit as part of an energy-boosting eating plan.

banana and strawberry smoothie

Packed with energy-giving oats and fruit, this smoothie makes a perfect start to the day.

2 bananas, quartered
250g/9oz strawberries
30ml/2 tbsp oatmeal
550ml/18fl oz/2½ cups natural
    live yogurt

Peel and chop the banana into large chunks; top the strawberries. Place the ingredients in a food processor or blender and process until creamy. Pour the smoothie mixture into tall glasses and serve.

plum and mango smoothie

150g/5oz fresh plums
300g/11oz mango
15ml/1 tbsp honey
550ml/18fl oz/2½ cups natural
    live yogurt

Stone (pit) the plums, peel and chop the mango into large chunks. Place the ingredients in a food processor or blender. Process for 1–2 minutes until frothy. Pour into large glasses and serve.

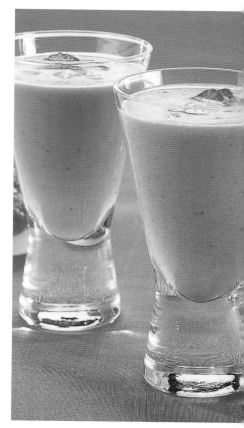

▲ *Experiment with combinations of your favourite fruits. For maximum nutritional content, serve smoothies immediately.*

21 aerobic exercise

Sustained by oxygen, aerobic exercises raise the heart rate for prolonged periods. They burn fat, boost the immune system and leave you with an energy surplus that increases general stamina.

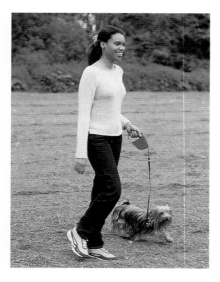

◄ *Aerobic exercise helps to increase and stabilize your stamina and energy levels.*

could alternate swimming with tennis. Remember to drink plenty of water when you exercise, as you can easily become dehydrated.

endless choice

Tennis, badminton, walking, jogging, cycling and swimming all offer excellent aerobic exercise – with the bonus being that they are inexpensive and enjoyable. Most gyms offer classes that use steps or weights, and some have tennis and badminton courts. Many offer dance classes in diverse styles as well. Choose an activity that matches your fitness level.

extra stamina

Aerobics will help give a real boost to your stamina and overall fitness levels. If you are feeling tired or frustrated, go for a walk or do some simple exercises for 10-15 minutes – note how energized you feel afterwards.

You should aim to do your chosen aerobics exercise for 45 minutes, three times a week, and it is a good idea to vary what you do, so that you don't become bored. For example, you

AEROBIC TIPS
• Choose an exercise that you enjoy: if you find the gym boring, try dancing, tennis or walking.
• Once you get started, the benefits will be such that you won't want to stop. Your mental outlook will improve as well: exercise helps to keep depression at bay.

42 / energizing treatments

22 anaerobic exercise

An exercise made up of short bursts of activity is called anaerobic. The muscles work intensely for short periods and, with continued exercise, they become stronger, providing you with more energy.

building strength

Muscle tissue is lost as the body ages, so it is important to begin building a strong physique as early as possible. And with physical strength comes confidence – a precious attribute that will see you through all of life's uncertainties. Strive to create an exercise regime that works for you, one that you can incorporate easily and enjoyably into your daily routine.

You can ask for advice on anaerobics at your local gym: many of the instructors are trained to offer an initial consultation on workouts and diet. Personal trainers offer a programme that is tailored to your own changing needs.

fighting fit

Before beginning a new anaerobics regime, check with your doctor if you have back or joint problems. Always do warm-up stretches, especially before using weights or playing squash, as cold muscles and ligaments can easily become strained.

Anaerobics result in the build–up of lactic acid in the muscles, causing temporary discomfort, which is why they cannot be sustained for long – lactic acid must leave the muscles before you can continue.

At the start of a new exercise, it is wise to limit yourself to 15-20 minutes a session, gradually increasing this as your strength increases. Always stop exercising if you are in pain.

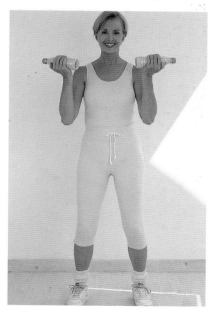

▲ *Anaerobic exercises help increase your energy levels by improving muscle mass.*

23

stimulating stretches

Chronic tension can easily lead to fatigue and exhaustion. When your memory and concentration suffer and stress leads to constant tiredness, these exercises may be helpful.

shoulder stand

1 Lie on your back, with your legs straight out and your arms by your side. Raise your legs until vertical. Continue lifting them over your head while raising your buttocks off the floor.

2 Supporting your lower back with your hands, slowly bring your back and legs to the vertical position.

3 Hold for a few moments, then return to the original position.

Caution: Avoid inverted position exercises if pregnant, and always seek medical advice if you suffer from high blood pressure or an overactive thyroid.

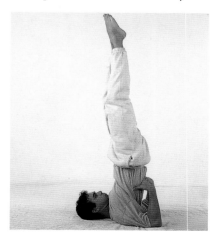

fish posture

1 Lie flat on your back.

2 Arch your back until the top of your head is resting on the floor. Hold the position, then relax.

Caution: This exercise is best avoided by those with neck problems.

leg clasp

1 Stand upright with your feet together. Bending forwards, clasp your hands behind your legs, as far down as is comfortable.

2 Steadily pull your head towards your legs. Go only as far as you can manage without strain. Hold for a few moments, then slowly uncurl and return to an upright position.

backwards bend

1 Stand with your hands on your hips, and your feet slightly apart.

2 Breathe in, then exhale as you bend backwards from the waist. Do not go further than is comfortable.

Caution: Avoid this stretch if you have any back problems.

◀ *Stretches bring blood to the brain and help boost your mental agility and mood.*

24 refreshing water sports

Sports that take place in or around water are, by their very nature, exhilarating. They range from the adventurous – sailing, water skiing, snorkelling, surfing and scuba diving – to healthy swimming.

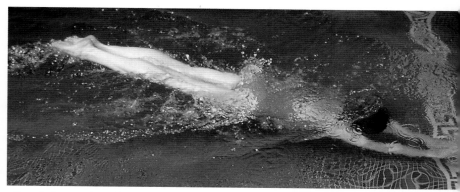

stimulating swimming

One of the most complete exercises you can do, swimming works all of the major muscle groups of the body without putting strain on the joints and spine – so people of all levels of fitness can enjoy the activity.

An exercise that is both aerobic and anaerobic, vigorous swimming also burns up anywhere between 500-700 calories an hour – so if you're trying to lose weight while you energize, this is a good choice. It will also raise your metabolism for several hours afterwards, meaning that you will burn more calories even at rest. To make the most of the activity, it is best to brush up on your strokes

▲ *Simple swimming is a great exercise, available at most local leisure centres.*

and make sure you have the proper form. If you paddle with your head above the water, you may be placing strain on your neck and shoulders, exacerbating back pain.

everyone in the water

It can be fun and invigorating to share exercise with a group. Classes in water aerobics, swimming and yoga are held at most pools, and some offer scuba diving as well. While on holiday, why not try snorkelling, or lessons in water skiing, sailing and surfing, all of which are challenging and rewarding.

25

energy-channelling t'ai chi

Practised by millions of Chinese, T'ai Chi Chuan combines exercise with meditation. Its emphasis is on channelling and helping the flow of energy, or "chi", rather than simply building physical strength.

cloud hands

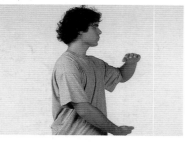

1 Begin with your right hand facing your navel, your left hand directly above it, facing your chest. Slowly turn your waist to the left, shifting your weight on to your left leg. At the same time, turn your palms towards each other, as if holding a large ball.

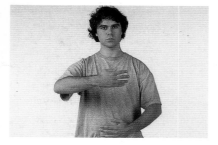

2 Bring your waist back to the front. As you do so, lower your left hand until it is opposite the navel and raise your right hand to the level of your chest, with your palms facing your body.

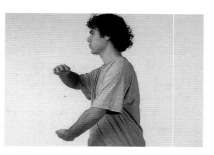

3 Now turn your waist to the right, shifting the weight across to your right leg, and turn your palms towards each other in a mirror image of Step 1. Repeat the sequence several times and note how it becomes more fluid.

26 mind-sharpening yoga

Yoga is one of the best ways to keep the joints and muscles flexible. It can relieve problems such as stress and anxiety, depression, back pain, asthma and insomnia – all of which can sap your energy.

the tree pose

To do this classical asana (yoga pose), stand with your feet hip-width apart, toes evenly spread. Allow your right leg to float up, bent at the knee. Take hold of your right foot and position the sole against the inner thigh of your standing leg, with the bent knee out to the side. If you cannot achieve this, place the sole where it is comfortable on the inside of the straight leg. Realign your pelvis, tucking your tailbone under, and softly fix your gaze on a point in front of you to help you balance. When you feel steady, raise your arms like the branches of a tree, breathing in. Hold the position for several breaths, and bring leg and arms down on an out-breath. Repeat with the opposite leg.

When you have worked both sides, stand with knees bent and drop the trunk forward and down, arms and head hanging loosely. This is excellent for neck exercises, as the weight of the head helps to extend the cervical spine. Move your head up gently, also breathing gently to loosen any tension. Uncurl your spine slowly and bring your chin up last, then rest.

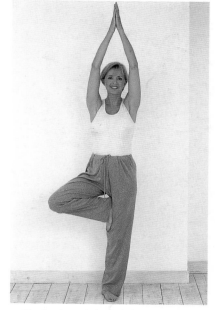

▲ *The best way to learn is from a teacher, but this exercise may be tried safely at home.*

TONING MUSCLES

Balancing poses sharpen the mind as well as exercising a lot of "inner" muscles. If balance is a problem, lean against a wall and experiment with the position of the bent leg.

27 uplifting oils

Aromatherapy treatments can be an effective means of restoring vitality and helping body and soul to recuperate after illness; citrus oils are very good at lifting moods and improving energy levels.

invigorating bath

Try this bath for a strong boost to the system, either in the morning or as a special afternoon reviving session.

4 drops of bergamot oil
2 drops of neroli oil
several drops of almond
   or wheatgerm oil

Fill the bathtub with warm water, then swirl essential oil drops in the bath just before getting in, so that their potency is at its height. Settle into the water and breathe in the stimulating scent.

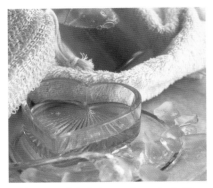

▲ Use essential oils to scent your bath oil.

▼ Use different scents around the home.

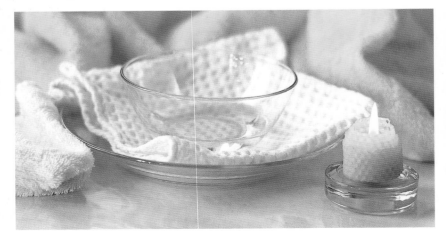

Imagine beginning your day by soaking in a refreshing bath filled with exotic flowers and spices.

Transport yourself to the midst of a pine forest, an oriental spice market or a citrus orange grove with just a few drops of essential oil.

invigorating bath oil

Herbal baths can be used for therapeutic purposes to raise energy levels and stimulate the senses. Simply scatter sprigs of herbs in the bath water or use their concentrated oil essences.

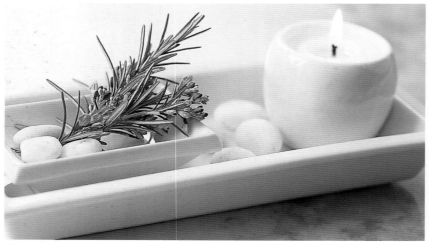

For a simple bath using essential oils, first draw the water and then measure out 5 drops. The oils form a thin film on the surface, and this, aided by the warmth of the water, will be partly absorbed by the skin.

**milk & honey
bath oil with rosemary**
The milk in this bath will leave your skin silky smooth.
2 eggs
45ml/3 tbsp rosemary oil
10ml/2 tsp honey

▲ *The heady scent of rosemary provides an immediate physical and psychological uplift.*

10ml/2 tsp baby or other
    mild shampoo
15ml/1 tbsp vodka
150ml/¼ pint/⅔ cup milk

Beat the eggs and oil together, then add the other ingredients and mix thoroughly. Pour into a clean glass bottle. Add 30–45ml/2–3 tbsp to the bath and keep the remainder chilled until ready for further use.

30 instant revitalizing massage

At any time of the day, energy levels can flag: after a meeting, when taking the children to school or out shopping. You can give yourself a quick "wake-up call" by doing this effective self-massage routine.

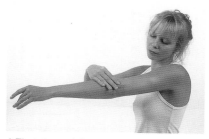

1 First, knead the arms, working rapidly from wrist to shoulder and back again with a firm squeezing movement. Next, rub swiftly upwards on the outside arm to stimulate circulation.

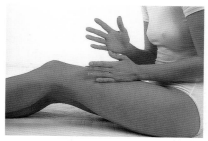

3 With the outside edge of the hands, lightly hack on the front of each thigh, using a rapid motion. Do not karate-chop the thighs – the hands should spring up from the muscles.

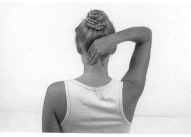

2 With the fingers and thumb of one hand, firmly squeeze your neck muscles using a gentle circular motion. Slowly work up the neck and then back down again. Continue the exercise until you feel the muscles have loosened.

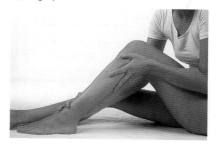

4 Now rub the calves vigorously to loosen them and get the blood flowing. It is best to do this with the knees bent. Work from the ankle to the knee, using alternating hands. Finally, stand up and shake your entire body, to let go of any stiffness and tensions.

re-balancing reflexology

Reflexology attempts to address imbalances in the body by applying pressure to corresponding points on the feet. The therapy encourages the healing and restoration of the body's equilibrium.

energy level enhancer

These simple reflexology exercises will help to stimulate the flow of energy through particular areas. Each section marked on the foot represents a different part of the body. Try the treatments on your own feet, or get a friend to help. Rest for a half hour after the treatment; your organs need time to readjust after stimulation.

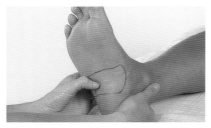

3 Work the small intestines to aid the uptake of nutrients.

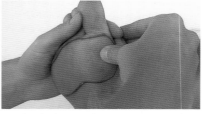

1 Work the lungs in order to improve your breathing.

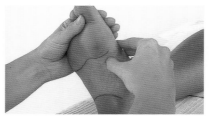

4 Work the whole digestive area: food is turned into energy during digestion.

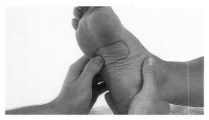

2 Work the liver; many of its functions are crucial to your health and stamina.

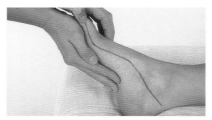

5 Work up and down the spine, the central column of your energy flow.

32 restorative flowers

Developed by Dr Edward Bach in the early 20th century, Bach flower remedies work on the premise that flower essences can enhance energy levels by restoring positive feelings and emotions.

Available from good-quality health food shops, Bach flower essences are sold separately. You can either ask your health practitioner to create tailor-made treatments for you, or try the following combinations:

exhaustion mix
Elm, Gorse, Hornbeam, Mustard, Oak, Olive, Walnut and Rose. This mix is useful as a pick-me-up after prolonged periods of work; it is also useful when responsibilities place a drain on the system.

confidence mix
Centaury, Chestnut Bud, Gentian, Larch, Pine, Sweet Chestnut, Walnut and Wild Rose. Helps to build inner confidence and constancy.

work stress mix
Gentian, Hornbeam, Impatiens, Mustard, Olive, Rock Water, Vervain, Walnut and White Chestnut. This mixture refreshes and restores interest when you are under stress at work. The Emergency Essence mix is also useful during stressful or anxious situations of any variety.

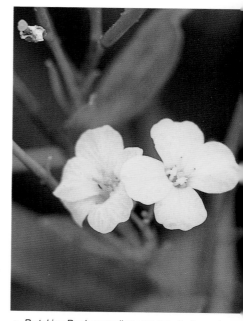

▲ By taking Bach remedies, you may find relief from stress and build up your inner resources, thereby energizing body and soul.

study and intuition mix
Cerato, Chestnut Bud, Clematis, Impatiens, Rock Water, Scleranthus, White Chestnut and Wild Oat. Helps with concentration during work and study, and boosts enthusiasm.

33 colour stimulants

Different colours can be used to stimulate and revive the senses, giving body and mind a real lift. Choose warm, vibrant shades for clothes, food and furnishings as part of your energizing strategy.

exhilarating wardrobe

For a reviving colour hit, choose clothes of red, orange and yellow hues, which are hot and stimulating. Red gives you extra energy and heals

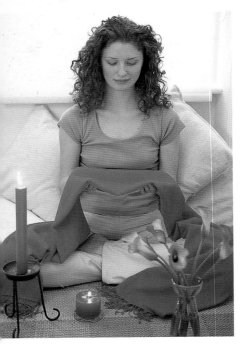

▲ Stimulating high-energy colours, such as red, orange and yellow, can help activate your passion for life.

lethargy and tiredness, while orange is said to create optimism and change, at the same time acting to heal grief and disappointment. To encourage more laughter, joy and fun in your life, and to keep depression at bay, opt for yellow clothes and accessories. Warm colours make your skin glow and work to attract other people, making you feel more vibrant and sociable.

happy interiors

Colour in the home or workplace can have a big impact on productivity. Paint the kitchen a glowing yellow to add cheer and inspire your cooking experience. Solid red or orange walls in a room can be overpowering, but you can easily splash accents of these hues in a room to increase mental alacrity. Spring green shades also have a livening effect.

mood foods

If you want to increase your zest for life, choose "passionate" foods – red strawberries and cherries, orange carrots and pumpkins, yellow peppers and squashes. Organic foods, grown without additives, are best.

34 energizing crystals

When the body is in a state of imbalance, a lack of energy is often felt. Correcting the balance using crystal techniques may help to restore and augment your physical stamina.

Red, orange and yellow crystals have the effect of promoting an increase in energy. Bright, strong colours – such as a deep-red garnet, golden amber or topaz – are very dynamic and stimulating. The more earthy tones of tiger's eye, citrine and jasper tend to foster an increase in practical motivation, so these are good to use when you need an energy boost for specific chores or projects.

You may find some of the stones too energizing at certain times. For example, golden citrine quartz is a wonderful substitute for the sun's warm energy – but on a hot summer's day, you might find it uncomfortable. Experiment with the stones, and soon you will know what each can do, and which is best for a particular situation.

QUICK FIX
To provide a quick burst of energy, recline comfortably and hold one clear quartz crystal – pointed upwards – in each hand. Place a large citrine at the solar plexus. Remain in position until you feel the stone's energy has "recharged" you.

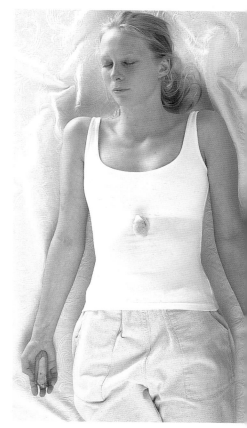

▲ During times of special need, you can give yourself an extra boost by using stones that directly stimulate vitality.

35

arousing bath oils

Effective treatments for dry skin, bath blends with uplifting essential oils can also have a beneficial influence on mood and health. The base oils in this recipe – almond and wheatgerm – are very gentle.

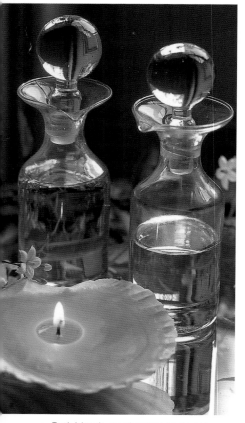

grapefruit and coriander bath oil
The combination of grapefruit and coriander has a wonderfully refreshing and arousing effect on the system, and the base oils soothe and calm flaky, dry skin. This blend is a potent reviver for times when you are recovering from a cold or flu.

100ml/3½fl oz/scant ½ cup almond oil
20ml/4 tsp wheatgerm oil
30 drops grapefruit essential oil
30 drops coriander essential oil
opaque glass bottle

Mix all of the ingredients in the bottle and shake well. Pour about 1 tbsp into the bath just prior to getting in and swirl to disperse. This recipe makes about 120ml/4fl oz/scant ½ cup.

CAUTION
When using citrus oils such as grapefruit, orange and lemon for the first time, try a small amount – the acids in citrus can sometimes irritate very sensitive skin. Always keep oils away from the eyes.

▲ Bath blends are simple to make at home and they are chemical-free – so you know exactly what you are putting on your skin.

reviving rose bath salts

Bath blends that contain a mixture of salts and aromatic flowers or herbs have long been used to treat a variety of complaints. Although many salts can be used, this blend uses simple sea salt.

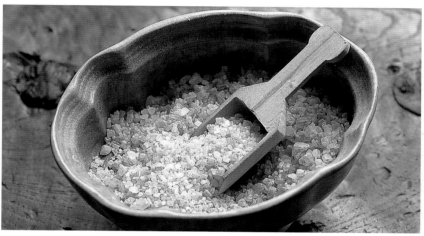

rose bath salts

10g/¼oz dried rose petals
mortar and pestle or electric
    coffee grinder
500g/1¼lb coarse sea salt
10 drops rose geranium essential oil
5 drops lavender essential oil
5 drops bergamot essential oil
decorative 500g/1¼lb glass jar,
    with close-fitting lid

Grind all but a handful of the rose petals (left whole for decoration). Mix the ground petals into the salt. Add the essential oils; stir thoroughly.

▲ *Soak in a bath of aromatic rose bath salts to scent the skin and lift the spirits.*

Spoon into the jar, adding a layer of whole rose petals halfway up. Place the lid on firmly and store in a cool, dry place. Makes about 500g/1¼lb.

how to use bath salts

Add 2 heaped tablespoons to running water in a medium–hot bath – if the water is too hot, the salt may elevate your heart rate and irritate your skin. Get in the tub and immerse yourself for a maximum of 15 minutes.

37 ginger body scrub

With its invigorating aroma and chemical action, ginger stimulates circulation, making it an excellent ingredient for an energizing body scrub. Clay and honey clean the skin by drawing out impurities.

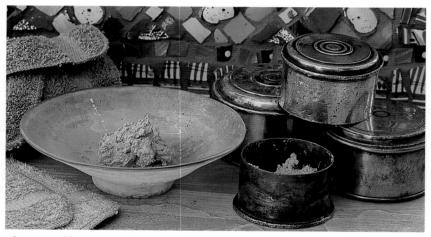

ginger and honey scrub
2 small bowls
20ml/4 tsp kaolin
10ml/2 tsp green clay
15ml/1 tbsp ground almonds
15ml/1 tbsp clear honey
30ml/2 tbsp warm water
15ml/1 tbsp orange flower water
3 drops ginger essential oil
small spoon
glass storage jar

In one bowl, place the kaolin, green clay and ground almonds. In the other, dissolve the honey in the water,

▲ *Rejuvenate your skin with a fresh scrub.*

and then add the orange flower water and essential oil. Slowly pour the honey, water, orange flower and oil mixture into the kaolin, clay and ground almond mixture. Blend the mixture using the spoon. To use, massage into the skin in a circular motion, adding a little water if necessary. Rinse off with warm water. It is best to use all the scrub in one treatment, but you can store the remainder in a glass jar in the refrigerator for up to 4 weeks.

38   tansy skin freshener

Tansy leaves have a strong, singular scent, and the plant is easy to grow. Pick fresh leaves for this invigorating skin tonic, and use it in the morning to give your skin a garden-fresh start to the day.

In ancient Greece, tansy was said to have been given to Ganymede to make him immortal. The herbalist Culpeper claimed it was a cure for diseases of the skin. Today, tansy's known tonic and stimulant qualities make it an ideal skin freshener.

tansy freshener
1 large handful of tansy leaves
150ml/¼ pint/⅔ cup water
150ml/¼ pint/⅔ cup milk
pan
strainer
jar

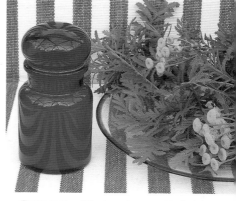

▲ *Tansy tonic will invigorate your skin first thing in the morning.*

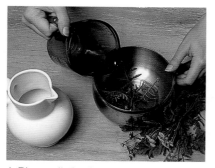

1 Place all the ingredients in a small pan and bring to the boil. Simmer for 15 minutes, then remove from the heat and allow to cool.

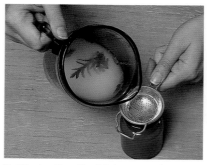

2 Strain the liquid into a glass jar. Store the tonic in the refrigerator and apply cold to the skin for a refreshing jolt of energy.

39

lemon verbena hair rinse

This rinse stimulates the pores and circulation of the scalp – and it bestows a wonderful, invigorating fragrance upon your hair. Use the fresh leaves of the lemon verbena plant for this recipe.

lemon verbena rinse
250ml/8fl oz/1 cup boiling water
1 handful of lemon verbena leaves
bowl
jug (pitcher)
strainer

Place the lemon verbena leaves in a bowl and pour the boiling water over. Set aside to infuse for at least one hour. Strain the liquid and discard the leaves. After normal washing and conditioning, pour the rinse over your hair, covering the strands and scalp. Dry and style as usual.

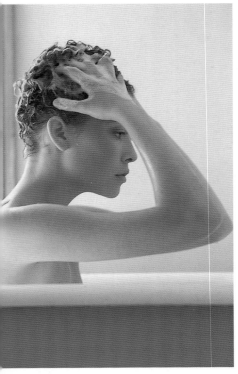

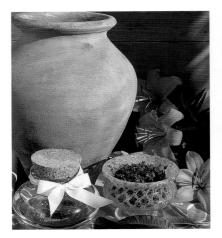

▲ *After shampooing, a herbal hair tonic can enhance circulation of the scalp, leaving it feeling tingling and refreshed.*

▸ *Lemon verbena has a multitude of uses and is easily grown in the garden.*

40 chakras for energy

You can increase your awareness of the energy "highway" that corresponds to the central nervous system by visualizing energy moving up and down the spine and passing through the chakras.

gestures for energy moving

By practising moving energy through the spine, eventually you will perceive these movements as actual rather than imaginary, and can start meditating on the qualities of the chakras. This will deepen your relationship with your senses.

2 Continue breathing in as you raise your hands slowly up the front of your body, "drawing" the energy up through the spine and into the love chakras in the heart area.

3 Continue, still breathing in, raising your hands and drawing the energy up through the throat area. Finish the breath in by taking your hands up past your face , spreading your arms wide and looking up. This is a joyful, exuberant movement.

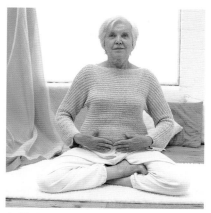

1 Sitting errect in a cross-legged position, bring your palms to face your lower abdomen with fingertips just touching. Start to breathe in, feeling that you are drawing vital energy up from the earth through the base of your body into the life chakras in the abdominal area.

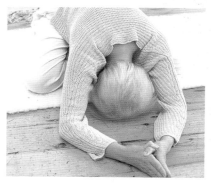

4 Now breathe out slowly as you lean forward to bring your head and joined hands to the floor in an attitude of relaxed and trusting surrender. Repeat the sequence once or twice more.

Step into a cold shower to provide a gentle shock to a sluggish system. You will feel instantly refreshed and wide awake.

42 go for a brisk walk

Walking is one of the simplest and most effective forms of exercise. It is a means of accelerating your physical energy levels and consequently raising your spirits – and it is enjoyable.

Walking at a fast pace provides many physiological benefits: it boosts your heart rate and respiration, speeds up your metabolism, tones your muscles and brings more oxygen to your bloodstream. It also causes the body to produce endorphins – the "feel good" hormones – which lift your mood and strengthen your immune system, helping to keep illness at bay.

meditation on the go
Walking can be a form of meditation, too. When you're feeling fed up or annoyed, get out into the countryside and into the fresh air. As you stride out, make your surroundings and the pleasure of the day the focus of your attention and try not to consider your own emotions. It is likely that your problems will begin to feel less acute and oppressive feelings will lift. It is almost as though the physical steps are mental steps that bring you closer to understanding difficult situations or overcoming obstacles.

▸ *Just taking a 10-15 minute walk can help you put any problems in perspective, and aid you in coming up with new solutions.*

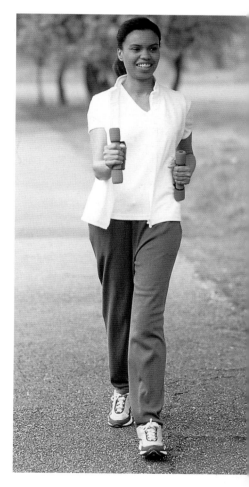

43 practise deep breathing

The power of proper breathing should not be underestimated – it oxygenates the blood, aiding thought processes and boosting physical energy. This simple technique can be carried out anywhere.

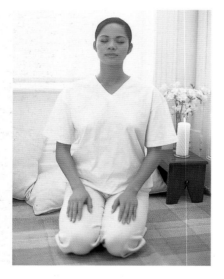

◄ *With regular practise, deep breathing can reduce stress on your nervous system.*

Many people do not breathe properly, taking shallow or quick gulps of air. By breathing from the diaphragm, you will bring oxygen all the way to the bottom of your lungs. This will improve your circulation, enhancing the body's systems and energy levels.

exercise and visualize

When practising deep breathing, there are many ways of concentrating the mind in order to heighten your physical stamina and mood, and to help quell the negative inner "voice" that can drain your reserves and dampen your spirits.

1 Start by counting your breaths, evenly, from one to ten.

2 Note the physical changes at the nostrils and the abdomen, as your breath moves in and out.

3 Notice the inner stillness as you change from exhalation to inhalation, from inhalation to exhalation. Now imagine drawing new energy into your lungs with each breath.

4 Close your eyes and conjure up an image that evokes a feeling of wholeness, joy and serenity. This could be a beautiful, natural scene with mountains or a valley, the undulating waves of the ocean, the sun's bright rays or a child you are fond of. Breathe in this complete image, until you feel its fresh, positive energy permeating throughout your entire body and mind.

5 Open your eyes and enjoy your feelings of renewed vigour.

44 inhale a scent

The sense of smell is the most primal of the five physical senses, and – although often played down in modern societies – it can be stimulated in many ways to evoke positive, invigorating feelings.

surround yourself with flowers

When feeling tired or low, give your mood an instant lift by buying a bunch of bright, luscious-scented flowers and placing them in a vase in a prominent place in your home or office. Choose from delicate freesias, roses and strong-scented star lilies; or daffodils, narcissi and hyacinths – which can be grown in pots indoors, in winter and spring. Fresh flowers certainly give you a boost.

evocative essential oils

Aromatherapy advocates using oil burners to disperse essential oils in a room. Place a few drops in the burner and light the candle beneath. Mints such as peppermint and spearmint are very stimulating, as are orange, geranium and ylang ylang. You can experiment with myriad different combinations of your favourite oils.

baking boost

The smell of baking bread or biscuits (cookies) can be a real mood booster – vanilla in particular triggers happy memories of childhood for many people. Choose a nutritious wholemeal

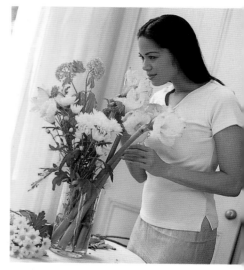
▲ Scent can trigger happy memories.

bread or biscuit recipe, and set to work – delicious aromas will soon waft through your house, putting a smile on your face.

refreshing air

Simply open a window to experience all the smells of grass, trees, blossoms, soil and rain outside. Even in winter, it can be very stimulating to let in the fresh air for just a few minutes.

45

eat a high-protein lunch

Do you often experience a mid-afternoon slump after eating a proper lunch? The cause may be foods that are high in fast-burning carbohydrates, leaving you with an energy deficit by around 3:00pm.

Many people's lives are too active to stop for a siesta during the afternoon; therefore, planning a lunch that provides sustaining energy through a busy working day is essential. Try a meal that includes high-protein chicken or tuna. Vegetarians may want to choose eggs, hummus or Quorn (mico-protein meat substitute), all of which are processed by the digestive system at a slower rate than carbohydrates and will provide energy for a longer period of time.

▼ *By choosing high-protein fish, you will feed your body with slower-burning fuel.*

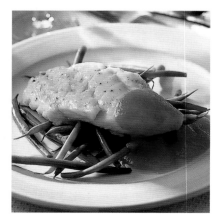

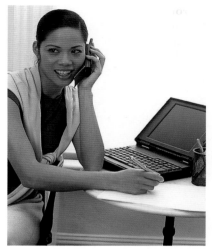

▲ *Eating a high-protein lunch will help to sustain you throughout the afternoon.*

protein snacking

When you do experience mid-afternoon hunger pangs, it's best not to reach for the biscuits (cookies) and chocolate – you'll be back in the same boat as before. These snacks are high in sugars that quickly disturb glucose levels, giving your body a rapid sugar rush, but leaving you feeling fatigued an hour later. Instead, grab a handful of nuts, or a rye cracker with cheese.

46 have a laugh

It has often been said that laughter is the best medicine. Research has confirmed this maxim: laughter raises endorphin levels, alleviating stress and allowing body and mind to work energetically.

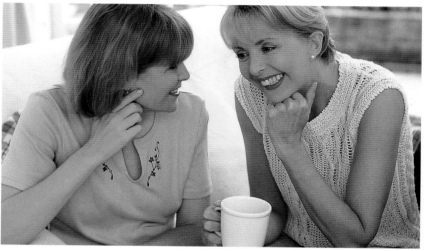

chuckle your way through the day
• Share a joke with a close friend or a group of friends, via talking, text messaging or email.
• Write down any funny thoughts that you may have and turn them into little stories. If you're good at drawing, make cartoons of the characters with captions.
• Try and see the silly side of serious or stressful situations: the best-adjusted people can laugh at most things, from disasters to death.
• Don't be afraid to laugh at yourself

▲ *People who laugh a lot are healthier overall. Fun is a very important aspect of life that should never be overlooked.*

and your own foibles. Everyone makes mistakes, and at least they can be enjoyed for their entertainment value in retrospect.

when feeling low key...
• Plan a night out at a comedy club with a group of friends.
• Watch videos of your favourite film or comedy series.

47 get up & dance

A highly aerobic activity, dancing wakes up the system in no uncertain terms – and it makes you feel great. Cares and worries quickly melt away after the first few minutes of a good boogie.

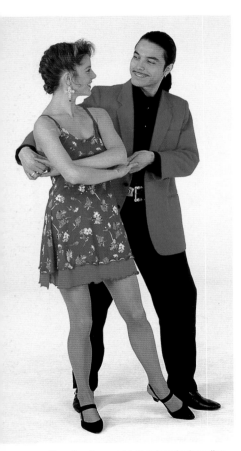

▲ *Dancing burns stress-related adrenaline and leaves you feeling wonderfully energized.*

Dancing has developed in all world cultures as a means of celebrating life. It is one of the most enjoyable ways to express yourself and to exercise. Many gyms offer classes in various styles: for example, salsa, samba, ceroc, jazz and ballroom. You may want to choose a highly vigorous dance form, such as rock 'n' roll; or perhaps choose one that is lower key, such as free-form or line dancing.

Some complex routines – such as those found in Indian and Indonesian classical forms – will keep your mind occupied with their intricate moves, and you will experience a real sense of accomplishment when you learn each sequence. Egyptian belly dancing is good for toning the midriff.

solo practice

Much enjoyment can be had by dancing with others, but you can also simply turn on your favourite up-tempo CD and dance by yourself, for a private workout guaranteed to enliven body and soul. If you are shy about dancing in public, this is the perfect prelude to going to a club with friends or signing up for a dance class.

48 think positively

Instead of concentrating on a daily catalogue of mishaps and frustrations or your own lack of luck, you can invigorate your life experience by looking on the bright side of everyday situations.

The power of positive thinking is so strong that it will help you overcome obstacles and create solutions to pressing problems. It will enable you to enjoy what you think and do, giving you new hope and energy.

life on the bright side

Negativity only serves to sap your inner resources. For example, if your car doesn't start in the morning and needs an all-day repair, it is easy to think your day is ruined. But looking on the positive side of the situation, you might just shrug your shoulders and say, "Oh well... this gives me a chance to work on a project at home today. I've been needing some time to myself..." In this way, you are not using up precious energy by allowing yourself to be ruled by anger and frustration – you are actually creating positive energy by seeing a challenge as an opportunity to do something enjoyable and rewarding.

Positive thinking can be applied to almost any scenario, enhancing your feelings of self-confidence and perhaps leading you to explore possibilities hitherto hidden.

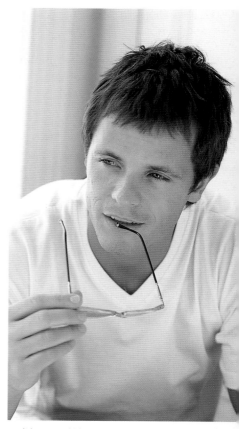

▲ *It is a good idea to start the day by "counting your blessings" – review all the good things you have, and go on from there.*

49 clear your mind

Feeling overwhelmed or bogged down with too much to do can lead to low energy levels at best, depression at worst. Clearing your mind of "excess baggage" can do wonders to improve your mood.

have a clear out

Sometimes a clear out of your physical environment can work wonders for your frame of mind. Set aside an evening to sort through old or unwanted clothes and get rid of them, giving them to friends or a charity shop. You will not only make way for new clothes, you will give yourself space for exciting new thoughts and feelings as well. In a similar way, you can clear a room or work space, creating more physical space and therefore more "head" or mental space in which to generate stimulating new ideas and solutions.

finishing projects

You may have so many tasks to complete in the course of a day, that your "to do" list becomes highly unmanageable. It is tempting to start something, then move on to the next "tick" in a panic. This will only frustrate and sap your energy, leaving you with a sense that nothing is ever completed. Try to create a reasonable list of tasks that you know you can accomplish, and do one thing at a time. Your list will magically diminish.

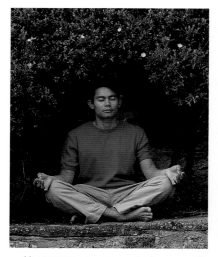

▲ *Use your energy economically – spend it on people and things that really matter.*

meditation time

Practising meditation is a pleasant way to energize, one in which you allow precious time and space for yourself. Meditation can help you to clear your mind of unwanted thoughts and feelings – perhaps some that have been holding you back for a long time. It can help you come to terms with situations and people over which you have no control.

50

have a good night's sleep

The value of sleep is too often underrated. To maintain our energy levels for the often hectic round of daily work, domestic and even leisure activities, a good night's sleep is essential.

Although we spend a third of our lives asleep, the importance of sleep is still something of a mystery. The body expends almost as much energy asleep as it does awake, and it is known that sleep is important for growth, learning and memory. Anyone who has suffered from insomnia will know that a lack of sleep causes irritability and poor concentration; if prolonged for greater periods, it can even cause ill health and hallucinations. A good night's sleep can be conducive to creativity – not only for artistic pursuits, but for the handling of the myriad daily tasks and challenges.

inspiring dreams

Many psychologists believe that dreams provide an important key to a person's mental and emotional health. It is thought that we work through problems and feelings when we dream, leaving us to wake with a fresh perspective. Dreams can also provide inspiration and insights, shedding light on intuitive knowledge and talents – and they can be highly enjoyable as a personal entertainment system, tuned in to our own "channel".

practical sleep aids

• Get plenty of exercise during the day, preferably out in the fresh air.
• Restrict coffee and tea to three cups a day; refrain from caffeine after 6pm.
• Take a warm – not hot – bath, about an hour before going to bed.
• Drink a cup of herbal tea or a hot, milky drink to soothe you to sleep.

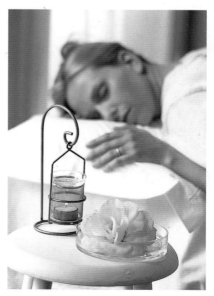

▲ *Create a peaceful bedroom atmosphere with soft lighting and soothing scents.*

detoxify

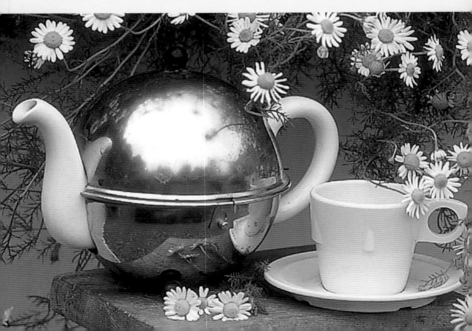

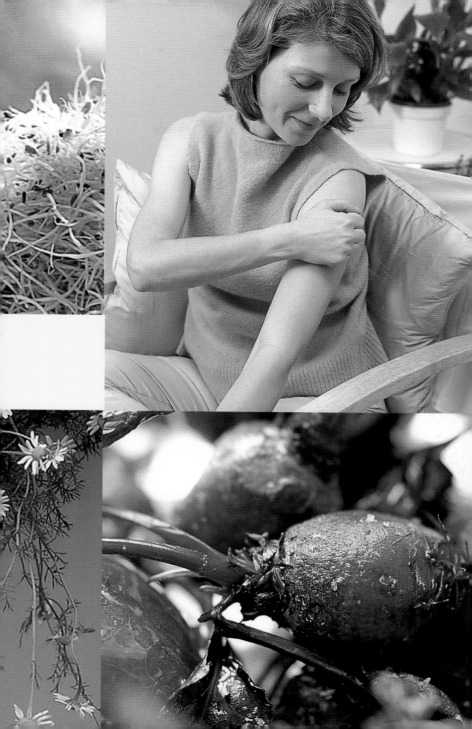

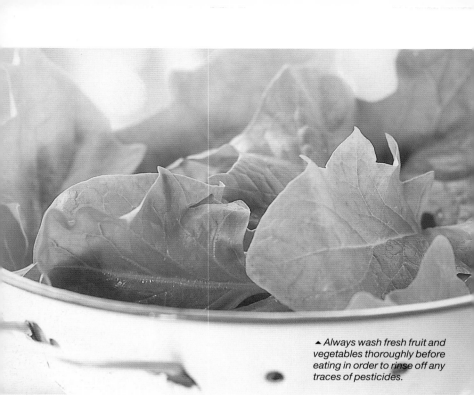

▲ Always wash fresh fruit and vegetables thoroughly before eating in order to rinse off any traces of pesticides.

learn to detox

In the course of our hectic lives, it is easy to overlook the longer term view of health. Under stress, we may succumb to bad habits such as smoking, drinking too much alcohol, eating too much or too poorly, and neglecting to exercise or sleep.

These factors, taken singly, may challenge the body so that its performance levels are low; two or more factors may have serious health implications over the years.

Sometimes it is a good idea to sit back and take stock of the situation. Perhaps you have had one too many colds or bouts of flu this season, or your energy levels have fallen, so that even simple, everyday routines have become something of a struggle?

Maybe you have become all too dependent on eating junk food instead of nourishing meals, and have noticed the pounds creeping up – or just a general dullness to your skin, hair and nails? Or perhaps you've stopped exercising and your fitness levels have fallen, leaving you feeling out of shape and depressed? You know you must do something to rectify the situation, but are unsure of where to begin. This chapter aims to help you make a fresh start.

detox diet

By following a brief detoxification programme, you can help to eliminate harmful substances from your body, clearing the way for a healthier lifestyle and new diet and fitness goals. A detox diet, which you can plan yourself, consists of eating only a few types of unprocessed food for a short period of time, while drinking plenty of water and herbal teas. This has the effect of flushing harmful toxins out of the system, restoring your energy levels and giving you a "clean slate".

For a brief introduction to detox, try a regime that lasts only one or two days. This will ease your body gently into a cleansed state, and is ideal in that it causes few side effects. A week-long detox is more intense and should be aimed at resolving more deeply embedded problems.

If at all possible, take the week off from work and responsibilities, as the change of food, drink and routine may leave you with temporary side effects. You may experience headaches, dizziness and stomach upset as toxins are washed out of your system, but they will subside once you begin to ease back into a normal, healthy diet.

essential exercise

Also crucial to any detox regime is exercise – it stimulates the lymphatic system, gets the heart pumping and improves circulation, removing waste matter and oxygenating the cells. Not only does exercise tone the muscles, it also acts to elevate your mood by releasing chemical substances called endorphins, which will help you to cope with stress more effectively, long after you have finished exercising. Choose from a range of aerobic exercises – those that push the heart rate up, such as cycling, running and dancing – and anaerobic exercises, those that help build muscle tissue and bone density through short bursts of activity. Examples of these

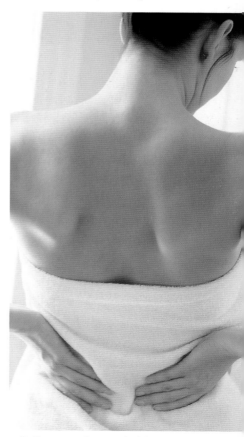

▲ Self-massage is a wonderful way to relax the body during detox, helping to ease tensions and release toxins from the cells.

are weight lifting and squash. Varying your routine will work all the muscle groups and keep you interested.

food for the soul

Relaxation and clearing the mind of negativity are just as important as physical exercise. The body and mind are fully linked – so stress, anger and negative thoughts can play havoc with your immune system, reducing its ability to eliminate toxins and making you more vulnerable to infections and disease.

By practising meditation and relaxation techniques for just 15–30 minutes a day, you will notice a marked improvement in your resilience to viruses, tension headaches and other stress-related illnesses. They will give you the ammunition to fight the daily battles that everyone is subject to – and savour life's pleasures even more.

With visualization techniques, it is possible to "rehearse" future stressful situations by imagining an important interview, for example, and then creating the conditions or solutions for a successful outcome. You can also explore what you really want from a relationship, friendships, job, home and family life.

alternative therapies

Like regular exercise, complementary therapies such as massage and aromatherapy have a beneficial effect on the lymphatic system, helping to flush out toxins. Massage has the added benefit of loosening tight muscles and helping to resolve chronic problems

▸ *Drink plenty of water throughout the day to keep you hydrated and to help your body flush out toxins.*

where tension is held in a certain area, such as the shoulders or abdomen.

Learn and practise self-massage techniques, and you will experience fewer problems with aching joints, neck tension and back pain. You can massage areas such as the face, hands and feet for an instant lift. Massaging the hands will also help you to avoid problems such as repetitive strain injury, a common hazard associated with manual and office work. Using aromatherapy oils in massage intensifies the experience.

Aim to look after your body now, and you will have less of a need to detox in the future. In addition, you will age in a more healthy way, with fewer of the complaints that beset many older people.

luxurious spa treatments

While you are following a detox regime, spa treatments such as saunas, mud wraps, body scrubs and baths will leave you feeling pampered and your skin feeling refreshed.

Saunas and wraps work by drawing impurities out of the skin, leaving the skin glowing. Other treatments such as facials, body scrubs and floral baths, are deep cleansing, mood enhancing and – best of all – enjoyable. Treat yourself by booking an appointment with a professional practitioner, or try one of the home-made treatments in this chapter.

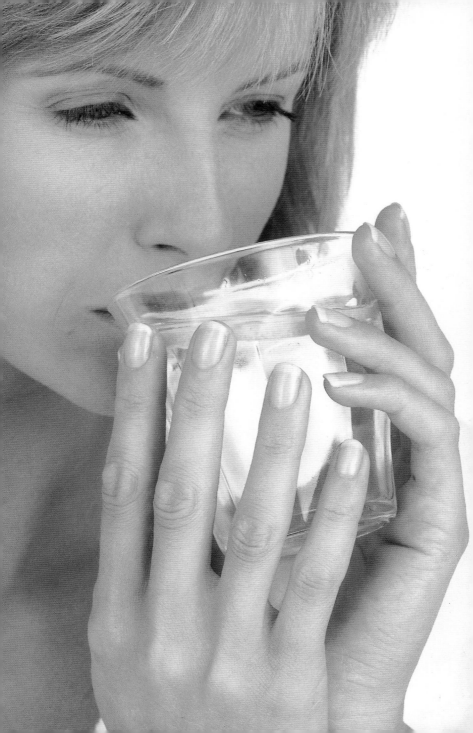

detox treatments

This chapter is organized so that you can choose the foods, detox plans, massage, exercises and treatments that will assist you on the road to a healthier body and a happier mind. Create a self-tailored detox programme by eating foods that will help your body to cleanse itself: fresh fruits and vegetables; tasty nuts and grains; soothing herbal tisanes and tangy smoothies. Decide on one of four detox plans, from a revitalizing 1-day detox to a 7-day detox – a sort of "spring clean". Massage techniques will address chronic problems – for example, aching shoulders or stiff neck – and chapters on exercise and meditation describe ways to recharge the batteries, both physically and mentally. Finally, pampering spa treatments – from invigorating body scrubs to floral-scented facials – will leave you cleansed, energized and looking as fresh and beautiful as you feel.

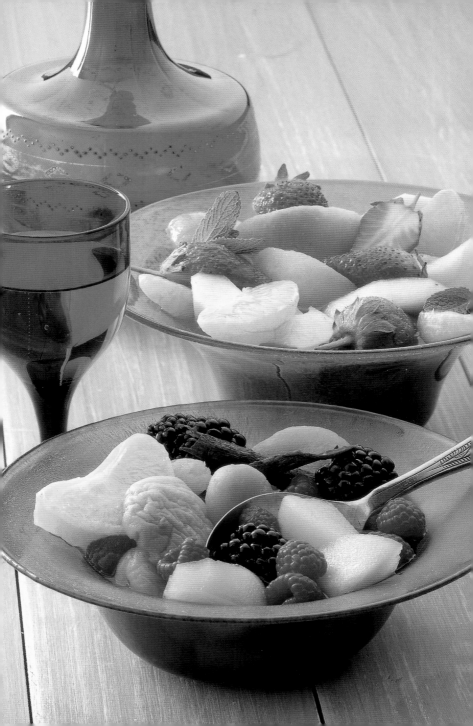

51 refreshing fruit

Fresh fruit is a storehouse of essential nutrients. Packed with vitamins, minerals, fibre, amino acids and enzymes, raw fruit should feature in any detox regime, as it helps bind and flush out toxins.

citrus fruits

These refreshing fruits are loaded with vitamin C, a powerful antioxidant that protects the body against harmful free radicals and inhibits premature aging. Antioxidants also help to reduce the risk of cancer and heart disease, and increase iron absorption.

Lemon is perhaps the best cleanser; its astringent and antiseptic properties stimulate the liver and gall bladder. A glass of hot water with freshly squeezed lemon juice is the ideal way to begin a detox day. Freshly squeezed oranges and grapefruits stimulate the digestion and tone the system. They are also an excellent source of betacarotene, calcium, phosphorus and potassium.

apples, pears and grapes

Crunchy apples contain malic and tartaric acid, which act to boost the digestive system and cleanse the liver. Their high pectin content binds heavy metals, such as lead. Apples also provide a steady stream of energy via fructose, a natural sugar.

When eaten regularly, pears help foster a good complexion and glossy

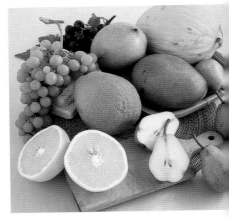

▲ The rich fibre and water content of tasty fruit make it the perfect internal cleanser.

hair. They are also an effective diuretic and laxative. Popular for one-day mono-diets, grapes are one of the most effective detoxifiers – in addition, they have been shown to relieve constipation and help kidney, liver, digestive and skin disorders. The white or red varieties are best.

mangoes

These fragrant soft fruits are reported to cleanse the blood. They also benefit the kidneys and digestive tract.

52 healthy dried fruit

Dried fruit provides plenty of sustaining energy and is invaluable in a detox regime. Although higher in calories than fresh fruit, unlike chocolate and sweets, dried fruit is a great source of nutrients.

Whenever buying dried fruit, look for unsulphured fruit, especially if you suffer from asthma. Choose from dried hunza apricots, figs, dates, raisins, apples, pears and peaches. Alternatively, you could opt for some more exotic fruits, such as pineapples, mangoes and papayas. These add tasty variety to your diet.

▾ *Perfect for snacks, dried fruit provides all the essential nutrients in a compact form.*

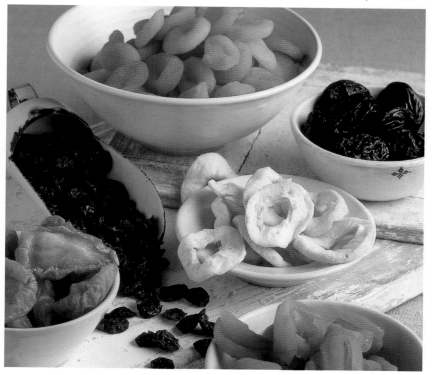

53 nutritious vegetables

The therapeutic benefits of fresh vegetables are due to an abundance of vitamins, minerals, bioflavonoids and other phytochemicals. Include plenty of different vegetables in your detox regime.

carrots

These root vegetables are highly beneficial. As well as cleansing, nourishing and stimulating the whole body, their abundant supply of betacarotene has been found to reduce the risk of cancer – eating just one medium-sized carrot per day can halve the risk of lung cancer.

garlic and onions

Containing antiviral and antibacterial nutrients, these vegetables are said to cleanse the system, fight cancer and lower blood cholesterol. Garlic boosts

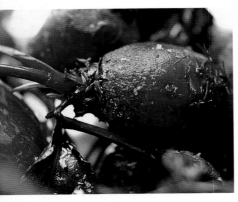

▲ *Beetroot (beet) is a good seasonal vegetable to include in your diet.*

the immune system and acts as an anti-inflammatory. Onions are best eaten raw, but their healing properties are not all lost through cooking.

beetroot

A powerful liver cleanser, beetroot (beet) is beneficial to the blood and a good laxative. It also has high levels of betacarotene, calcium and iron.

cruciferous family

Members of this family – including broccoli, Brussels sprouts, cauliflower, cabbage and watercress – are all among the detox superfoods. They stimulate the liver and supply a cancer-fighting cocktail of phytochemicals.

Broccoli also offers a plentiful supply of many B and C vitamins, in addition to minerals such as calcium, folic acid, iron, potassium and zinc.

spinach

A vast supply of antioxidants makes raw spinach an excellent choice for a detox diet. It contains betacarotene, vitamin C, calcium, folic acid, iron, potassium, thiamin and zinc. Young spinach makes a tasty addition to salads.

54 detox vegetable stock

Vegetable stock is used to add flavour to dishes such as soups and stews. Purchased stock is usually very high in salt, and should not be used in detox, as salt increases water retention.

veggie deluxe stock
15ml/1 tbsp sunflower oil
1 potato
1 carrot
1 celery stick
2 cloves of garlic (peeled)
1 sprig of thyme
1 bay leaf
few stalks of parsley
600ml/1 pint/2½ cups of water
freshly ground black pepper

1 Scrub, trim and chop the vegetables. Heat 15ml/1 tbsp sunflower oil in a large saucepan. Add the potato, carrot and celery, all chopped up into small pieces.

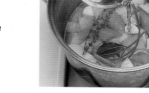

2 Cook them, covered, for 10 minutes until soft. Stir in the garlic, thyme, bay leaf and parsley. Pour the water into the pan and bring the mixture to the boil.

STOCKING UP
Larger quantities of stock can be made and stored in the freezer, or in the refrigerator to be used within 4 days.

3 Simmer the mixture, partially covered, for 40 minutes. Strain, and then season with freshly ground pepper. Use the vegetable stock as required in cooking.

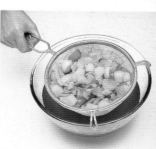

55 fantastic fibre

Not only are whole grains and cereals an excellent source of low-fat protein, they contain complex carbohydrates, fibre, vitamins and minerals to keep you energized during detox.

world of grains

Grains have been a part of the human diet for thousands of years, and have been cultivated for centuries. It is good to include a selection of different grains in your detox plan, including brown rice, barley, millet, oats, couscous, buckwheat and quinoa. Brown rice is used to treat digestive disorders, calm the nervous system and reduce the risk of bowel cancer. Oats absorb impurities in the blood, leaving the complexion glowing. The South American grain, quinoa, contains more protein than any other – about 14 per cent.

essential fibre

Unprocessed whole grains contain both soluble and insoluble fibre, both of which are fundamental in the prevention of constipation, colon and rectal cancers, ulcers and heart disease. Foods rich in fibre bind with harmful cholesterol and help it to pass through the body for elimination.

wheat warning!

Although nutritionally viable in its whole form, wheat is also a common allergen – it can irritate the body's ability to absorb some nutrients, and should be avoided during detox.

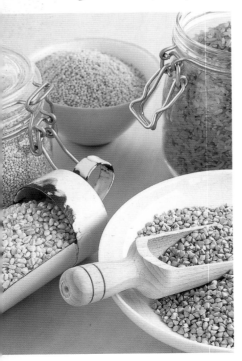

◄ *The starch in grains is absorbed slowly, keeping blood sugar levels even – important when you may be eating less than usual.*

56 vital pulses

Providing low-fat protein, fibre and vitamins, beans and pulses have long been a staple of vegetarian diets. They are bursting with minerals, including folate, iron, magnesium and potassium.

bean choice

It is preferable to use dry beans in cooking, as processing adds sugar and salt. The night before beginning a detox programme, try eating a nutritious stew or thick soup made from tasty lentils, dried peas, pinto and mung beans, or chickpeas.

bean feast

Most dried beans need to be soaked for at least 8 hours prior to using them in a recipe. To prepare, leave them overnight with plenty of fresh cold water. The next morning, drain and rinse the beans before boiling hard for at least 10 minutes, then leave them to simmer until they are fully cooked. (Note: lentils do not need to be soaked, nor boiled rapidly.)

Alternatively, follow a recipe for cooking instructions. Never eat beans raw or partially cooked, as they may cause an allergic reaction. When using a new bean, taste a small amount first, in case you are sensitive to it.

▶ *Studies show that eating just half a cup of cooked beans regularly reduces cholesterol levels by 20 per cent.*

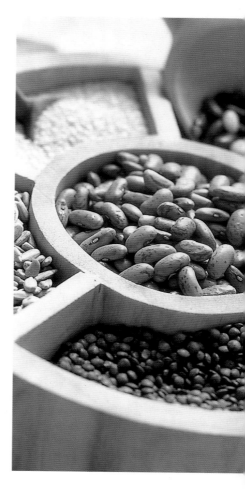

57 supersprouts

When beans, seeds and grains sprout, their nutritional value soars making them excellent detox ingredients: their vitamin C content rises by 60 per cent, and B vitamins by 30 per cent.

grow your own

It is simple to grow delicious sprouts. Commercial sprouter packs are available from health food stores, and they can be easily grown at home. Try the following:

Take a large, wide-mouthed jar and wash thoroughly. Place 15ml/1 tbsp of alfalfa seeds, soy, mung or other beans in the jar.

Cover the mouth of the jar with a clean piece of muslin (cheesecloth) or finely-woven mesh, and fasten tautly with an elastic band or a clean piece of string. Rinse the beans or seeds thoroughly in cold water, shaking off the excess. Place the jar in a darkened cupboard, and rinse the beans once or twice a day, as before.

The beans should sprout and be ready to eat in approximately 4–5 days. Once they are fully sprouted, refrigerate your supersprouts. You can keep a ready supply by beginning new jars on successive days.

➤ *Sprouts supply rich amounts of protein, vitamin E, potassium and phosphorus – all packaged in an easily digestible form.*

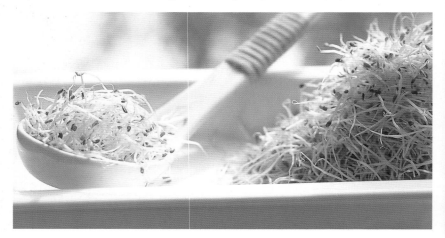

Packed with vitamins, minerals and **antioxidants,** seaweeds – such as arame, kombu, hijiki and wakame – improve the **condition** of your **skin**, hair and nails.

59 beneficial nuts & seeds

As an excellent alternative to meat and cheese choose protein-rich nuts and seeds when you embark on a detox. Their vitamin E content improves the skin, hair and nails.

nutty choice

Walnuts, almonds, cashews, hazelnuts and peanuts offer some of the best health benefits – they can be eaten on their own, or added to porridge, breads, casseroles and salads. Since they are a high-fat food, nuts should be eaten in moderation.

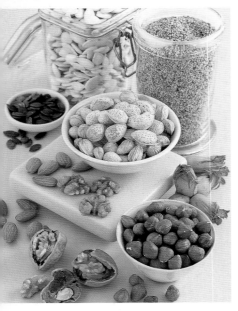

▲ Nuts are packed with B vitamins, iron, calcium, magnesium and potassium.

Seeds such as pumpkin, sunflower and sesame offer similar nutritional values with slightly fewer calories. Buy them in small quantities, seal and store in a cool place. Wholegrain toast spread with tahini (crushed sesame seed spread) makes a tasty and nutritious start to the day.

nutty oat snack

30ml/2 tbsp sunflower oil
30ml/2 tbsp honey or maple syrup
600g/21oz jumbo oats
50g/2oz sunflower seeds
50g/2oz pumpkin seeds
50g/2oz roughly chopped almonds,
   hazelnuts or unsalted peanuts
50g/2oz chopped dried apricots
   or raisins

Preheat oven to 150°C/300°F/Gas 2. In a large pan, heat the oil and honey until the mixture is thin. Stir in the remaining ingredients, except the apricots, until the dry ingredients are coated evenly. Spread the mixture on a baking sheet and toast for 30 minutes, until it turns light golden brown. Remove from the oven and stir in the apricots. Store in an airtight container.

60

fresh herbs

Herbs have a cleansing effect on the system, easing indigestion, nausea and constipation; they may also help to alleviate headaches and respiratory problems.

Although herbs are low in nutritional value they have a high concentration of essential oils, many of which are antioxidant, antiviral and antibacterial.

cooking herbs
Some of the most useful herbs for cooking delicious detox meals are also the most common. Look for fresh coriander (cilantro), basil, dill, mint, parsley, sage, rosemary and thyme. Many grocery stores and nurseries sell growing plants – fresh is best.

SUPER HERBS
The following cleansing herbs can complement your detox programme. Always consult a qualified naturopath before taking them for the first time.

MILK THISTLE – increases liver efficiency.
ECHINACEA – boosts the immune system.
GOTU KOLA – diminishes cellulite.
GOLDENSEAL – aids digestion and is antibacterial.
DANDELION – a gall bladder and liver tonic.

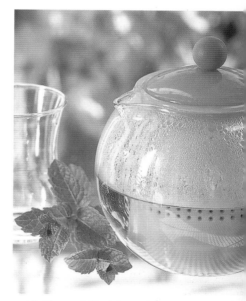

▲ Mint is a useful herb for easing nausea, indigestion and respiratory problems.

soothing mint tea
This tea is useful for your detox plan – it will settle stomach upsets and clear your sinuses. Place 10ml/2 tsp of fresh peppermint or spearmint leaves in a pot and add boiling water. Cover and leave for about 10 minutes to infuse, then strain and drink.

61

stimulating spices

Revered for their medicinal properties for thousands of years, spices are also a culinary mainstay. When added to dishes and drinks, they tend to have a stimulating and antiseptic effect on the body.

detox spice rack

Useful spices to include in your detox plan include fenugreek, nutmeg and turmeric, as they cleanse the body and help to release toxins. Cinnamon is also an effective cleanser; cardamom calms indigestion, as does coriander.

Cloves contain both antiseptic and anaesthetic qualities – clove oil has traditionally been used for toothache. Pepper is the most commonly used spice in the West. Black and white pepper aid digestion and help dispel wind, and cayenne promotes

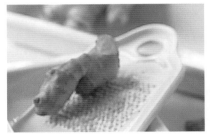

▴ *Add grated ginger to salads and stir-fries.*

sweating and the release of toxins through the skin (but is best used in small amounts only).

ginger

Fresh root ginger is one of the most powerful healing spices to include in a detox diet. Not only does it treat gastro-intestinal complaints and nausea, it also reduces the risk of some cancers. Add to stir-fries or grate into salads. You could also try this soothing tea: take two or three fine slices of ginger and place in a mug; add boiling water and infuse for 5-10 minutes. Add a teaspoon of honey if desired.

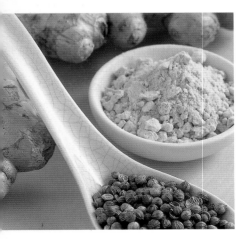

◀ *Fresh root ginger, fenugreek and coriander seeds are powerful system cleansers.*

62

relieving oils & vinegars

Oils provide essential fatty acids and vitamin E, both beneficial for the heart and skin. Cold-pressed oils are most nutritional. Cider vinegar is best for detoxing – it relieves headaches and aching joints.

wide choice

Organic olive, sunflower, safflower and grapeseed oils are all beneficial. Speciality oils such as walnut, sesame, almond and hazelnut are a tasty alternative. Almond oil is also good for massaging and moisturizing your body – it is easily absorbed into the skin.

Because oils are a high-calorie fat, it is important to use them in moderate amounts only during the latter days in a week-long detox diet. Wine vinegars should be avoided in detox, as they contain acetic acid, which hinders digestion.

sesame ginger dressing

120ml/4fl oz/½ cup cider vinegar
15ml/1 tbsp grated fresh root ginger
120ml/4fl oz/½ cup water
250ml/8fl oz/1 cup sunflower oil
10ml/2 tsp honey
15ml/1 tbsp sesame seeds

Place the vinegar in a bottle or jar. Add the grated ginger and allow to soak for 30 minutes. Add the water, oil, honey and sesame seeds. Shake well and add to green or fruit salad.

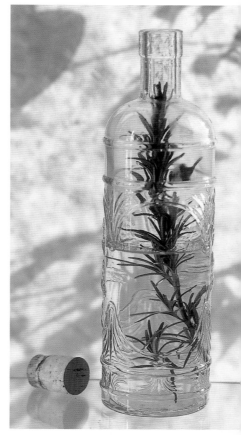

▲ *Use herbs, such as rosemary, to make tasty aromatic oils for salad dressings.*

63 hydrating water

Water is a vital nutrient that cannot be stored in the body. It is lost constantly through sweat, urination, defecation and exhaling vapour when you breathe. Aim to drink at least 1.5 litres/2½ pints each day.

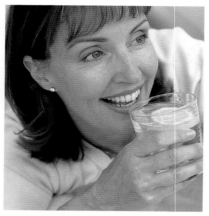

stay hydrated

Pure water – mineral or filtered tap water – will flush toxins from your organs. Diluted fruit and vegetable juices are also good choices. Avoid soft drinks containing sugar and preservatives as these place stress on your body and add sodium and empty calories. Carbonated water is acceptable, but drink it only in small amounts – dieticians believe that it raises the pH level in the stomach, making it harder for the body to digest protein.

▸ *Ice-cold water with a slice of lemon will boost your metabolism and burn calories.*

◂ *A cup of hot water with a slice of lemon is a refreshing and cleansing tonic.*

monitor your intake

It is a good idea to drink a large glass of water when you wake up in the morning, as your body dehydrates during the night, especially during warm or hot weather. It is best not to rely on your sense of thirst to tell you when to drink: keep sipping it throughout the whole day.

Most people do not drink enough fluids during the day, and this becomes noticeable when the urine turns a tell-tale dark amber colour. A pale golden colour means that you are probably taking in enough hydrating fluids.

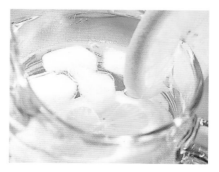

64 soothing herbal teas

Herbal teas offer medicinal benefits and, as drinks, have the advantage of hydrating the body. Unlike black teas and coffees, which contain caffeine, they do not strain the cardio-vascular system.

digestive tea

The fennel and caraway seeds in this tea aid digestion. It can be taken as a pleasant drink after a heavy meal or to soothe an upset stomach.

Put 5ml/1 tsp fennel and 2.5ml/½ tsp caraway seeds into a pot, adding 600ml/1 pint/2½ cups of boiling water. Steep for 10 minutes and serve with a dollop of honey.

bedtime tea

For a relaxing and calming tea to ease you to sleep, place 5ml/1 tsp chamomile, 2.5ml/½ tsp of valerian and 5ml/1 tsp of peppermint into a pot and infuse. Strain, add honey if desired, and drink. This is best taken 30 minutes to 1 hour before bedtime.

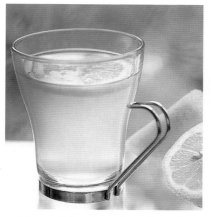

▲ A tea made from lavender and vervain helps ease the effects of overindulgence.

morning–after tea

This is a good liver reviver to take following a party or late night out. Sip it throughout the day until you feel your body and mind are refreshed. Place 5ml/1 tsp vervain and 2.5ml/½ tsp lavender flowers into a pot. Add 600ml/1 pint/2½ cups of boiling water, cover and steep for 10 minutes. Strain, add lemon and sweeten with honey.

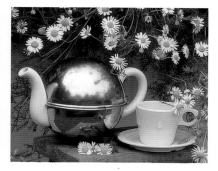

◄ Chamomile is a herb with calming, relaxing properties, perfect for bedtime.

65

flower tisanes

Teas made by steeping fresh sprigs of flowers in boiling water are called tisanes. Many blossoms can be used, such as chamomile, dandelion, lavender, rose, lime blossom, jasmine and bergamot.

lemon verbena tisane

This refreshing, lemon-flavoured tisane is delicious when enjoyed either hot or cold.

Take a flowering spray of lemon verbena (with a few leaves) and put in a cup. Add boiling water and steep for 4 minutes, when the tisane should be a pale golden colour. Remove the flowers and foliage, and add a small dollop of honey, if desired.

lime blossom tisane

This pale yellow tisane has been used traditionally to promote a good night's sleep; it is surprisingly creamy.

▼ The fragrance of tisanes, such as lime blossom, acts as a mood enhancer.

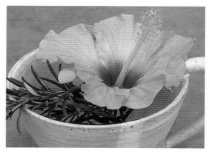

▲ Hibiscus flowers make a visual treat, as well as a soothing hot drink.

Pick lime flowers when they begin to open, using five or six for each cup. Add hot, not boiling, water and steep for 3–4 minutes. Remove the blossoms. Strain and drink with a slice of lemon.

hibiscus and rosemary tisane

With their flamboyant colouring, exotic hibiscus flowers make a dramatic and colourful tisane, enhanced with savoury rosemary.

Place one hibiscus flower and one rosemary sprig per cup and add some boiling water. Infuse for 4 minutes, removing the rosemary but leaving the hibiscus in place. Drink hot or chilled. Sweeten with honey.

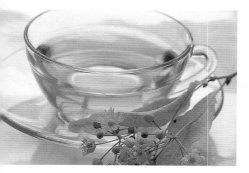

66 rejuvenating juices

Fresh fruit and vegetable juices play a vital role in detoxing – they stimulate the whole system and encourage the elimination of toxins. Drink juices fresh, as processing reduces nutritional values.

purple pep
For a healthy dose of antioxidants, try this rich, colourful juice.
3 carrots
115g/4 oz beetroot (beet)
30g/1 oz baby spinach
2 celery sticks

Scrub and trim the carrots and beetroot, then cut the beetroot into large chunks. Juice all the vegetables in a juice extractor, then pour into a glass and drink immediately.

citrus shake
This refreshing juice gently boosts the immune system.
1 pink grapefruit
1 blood orange
30ml/2 tbsp lemon juice

Peel the grapefruit and orange and cut into rough segments. Juice the fruit, then stir in the lemon juice.

juicing tips
• Drunk in the morning, fruit juices are useful for scouring waste products from the digestive tract.
• Vegetable juices are best drunk in the afternoon, as they re-establish the acid and alkaline balance of the body, giving a rejuvenating effect.
• Do not drink fresh juices if you suffer from health problems such as candida, diabetes or bowel disorders.

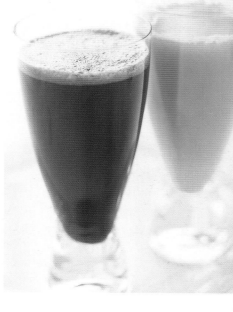

▼ *Purple Pep, an antioxidant powerhouse, and tangy and cleansing Citrus Shake.*

67

delicious smoothies

A blend of soft fruits and milk or yogurt, smoothies offer a tasty alternative to eating fruit. Their vitamin content makes them ideal detoxifiers. Summer smoothies can be partially frozen for a cool treat.

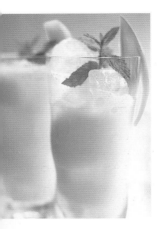

banana and mango smoothie

125g/4½oz banana
125g/4½oz mango
120ml/4fl oz/½ cup yogurt
　 or milk

Peel and chop the banana and mango into large chunks. Place the fruit in a food processor or blender with the yogurt or milk. Process for 1-2 minutes, until smooth and creamy, and pour into a large glass.

Add a sprig of mint for a tasty bite.

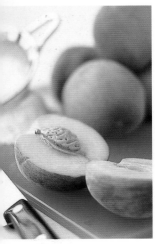

peach and blueberry smoothie

150g/5oz fresh peaches
150g/5oz blueberries
120ml/4fl oz/½ cup yogurt
　 or milk

Stone (pit) the peaches and chop the flesh into large chunks. Drop the peaches and the blueberries into a blender and add the yogurt or milk. Process for 1-2 minutes until the mixture turns frothy, then pour into a large glass and serve.

Substitute raspberries or strawberries for the blueberries. Frozen berries may be used when fruit is out of season.

68 food & drinks to avoid

Diet is the key to a fit body and a lively mind. Poor eating habits suppress the body's efficiency, and the following should be excluded during detox – ideally, they should always be kept to a minimum.

processed foods

Many modern food production methods overprocess foods, leaving nutritional values diminished – fibre, minerals and vitamins are stripped away, and an excess of sugar, fats and salt are added. Commercial farming and storing methods also add harmful chemicals and preservatives. Buy fresh organic foods whenever possible.

alcohol

The occasional glass of wine does little harm, and may even help prevent heart disease. Drunk in large amounts, however, alcohol damages the liver, depletes vitamin stores and dehydrates the system.

caffeine

Found in coffee, tea, chocolate and soft drinks, caffeine is a powerful stimulant that raises blood pressure and exacerbates nervous conditions. Before starting a detox diet, reduce caffeine consumption gradually to avoid withdrawal symptoms.

▸ *Eliminate cakes and biscuits, which are high in refined sugars, during a detox diet.*

dairy products

Butter, cheese and milk are high in unsaturated fats; these tend to slow down the lymphatic system, which is responsible for removing toxins from the body, so avoid when detoxing.

fish and meat

Meat is difficult to digest and, unless it is organic, may contain traces of growth hormones and preservatives used in production. Fish may contain pollutants, unless caught in deep seas.

salt and sugar

Excess salt overloads the kidneys and leads to water retention. Herbs or lemon juice are good substitues. Refined sugars can upset the body's sugar balance. Natural sugars in fruits and honey are kinder on the system.

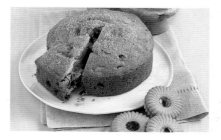

69 mono-diet detox

Based on eating just one type of raw fruit or vegetable, a 1-day mono diet is an excellent introduction to detoxing that will have a noticeably positive effect on your health and vitality levels.

the diet

Choose one type of organic vegetable or ripe fresh fruit. You will need 1.6kg/3½ lb of either: grapes, apples, pears, pineapple, papaya, carrots, cucumber or celery. Eat small meals and vary the way you prepare the food. For example, you could grate

▾ *After a 1-day mono diet, moving on to longer programmes will be simple.*

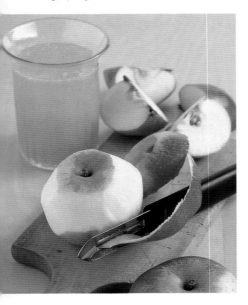

your chosen fruit or vegetable for breakfast, juice it for lunch and eat it whole for dinner.

In the morning, drink a cup of hot water with the juice of a half a lemon to kick-start the liver. It is important to drink at least 1.5 litres/ 2½ pints/6¼ cups of still mineral water, or filtered tap water, at intervals throughout the day.

vital exercise

• Morning: Practise simple stretches to stimulate your lymphatic system. Later in the morning, have an aromatherapy or a shiatsu massage, or try relaxation techniques such as deep breathing.
• Afternoon: Try some gentle yoga or Pilates exercises, or go for a swim, cycle or take a walk.
• Evening: Wind down by meditating or practising a simple visualization technique. Pamper yourself with a pedicure or manicure, read a book or listen to some calming music. Later, soak in an Epsom salts bath and prepare for bed early, perhaps relaxing with a good book or drinking a soothing herbal tea.

70

weekend detox

The 2-day detox plan is based on fruit and vegetable dishes and juices. Perfect for a quiet weekend, this is a gentle and effective detox that will give your digestive system a break.

the diet

• Morning: Kick-start your liver with a cup of hot water and lemon juice. For breakfast, prepare a fruit juice and dilute with water. Eat a small bunch of grapes or an apple mid-morning.
• Afternoon: Prepare a vegetable juice and a large salad for lunch, for example, tomatoes, cucumber, fennel, carrot and beetroot (beet). Drink plenty of water, either bottled mineral or filtered tap water.
• Evening: Have a dinner consisting of very lightly steamed vegetables, sprinkled with fresh herbs and lemon juice, along with some brown rice.

vital exercise

Take gentle exercise, such as yoga or Pilates, and do simple stretches all day. Walking or cycling will give you energy in the afternoon. It is a good idea to end each day with relaxation techniques or meditation.

don't detox:

• Directly after a bout of flu.
• If you have had liver disease or kidney failure; ask your doctor about diet.
• When under great stress; ie pressure at work, moving house, during a bereavement or after a divorce.
• If you have a serious medical condition or are taking prescription drugs for any reason.
• If you are pregnant or diabetic.
• If you are recovering from alcohol or drug addiction.

▼ Eating mainly vegetables and fruit allows the body to focus on eliminating toxins.

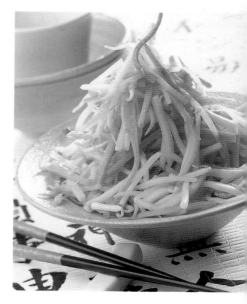

71

7-day detox

This rigorous plan is designed to provide a slow and steady detox. The plan combines and supplements the mono and weekend plans. Begin on a Friday, as the first few days are more intense.

the plan

• Day before: Ease into detox by including light, cleansing foods in your meals.
• Day one: Follow the guidelines for the 1-day mono diet.
• Days two and three: Follow the guidelines for the weekend detox. In the evening, have a sitz bath.
• Days four and five: Repeat days two and three, but include a fruit salad with yogurt for lunch and a baked potato with tofu or hummus for dinner. From day four, include snacks such as pumpkin seeds, dried fruit or nutty oat snack.
• Days six and seven: Repeat days four and five, including dried fruit steamed with fresh ginger. Add more protein to your meals, eg a grain or bean salad, lentil dahl or brown rice risotto. For dessert, eat live natural yogurt with a spoonful of honey. In the evening, take an Epsom salts bath to help flush out toxins.
• Days after: Slowly return to a healthy, varied diet based on nourishing, cleansing foods. Try not to overexert yourself, and avoid stressful situations, if at all possible.

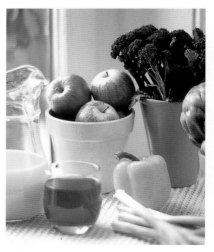

▲ The 7-day detox includes healthy, natural foods to help cleanse your system.

side effects

When following a detox programme, side effects are natural; their severity will depend on how many toxins are present in the system and how long your diet lasts. You may experience fatigue, headaches, nausea, chills, bad breath, furry tongue and irritability. Avoid painkillers; instead, drink plenty of water and herbal teas to aid the flushing out process.

72 hangover detox

If you have drunk too much alcohol, this hangover detox will ease the pain. The ideal is to consume a moderate amount in the first place, but the occasional overindulgence can be dealt with.

intake plan

Alcohol dehydrates your body, so keep sipping water all day. Although you may crave coffee and tea, caffeine acts as a diuretic – counter-productive when you are trying to rehydrate. Instead, try herbal teas with a little honey. To help settle your stomach and raise your blood sugar levels, eat a breakfast of natural muesli with yogurt and fruit, or a big bowl of porridge. For lunch, choose a light, filling meal that is low in fat – for example, a vegetable stir-fry with brown rice or couscous. At dinner time, a piece of baked fish or chicken with a salad, or a baked potato with salad are good choices.

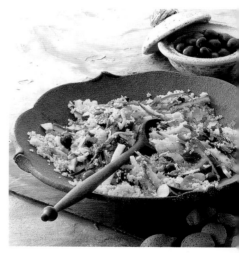

▲ Prepare a low-fat nutritious lunch to settle your stomach and set you on the road to recovery.

relax

You are bound to feel under par, so be kind to yourself. End the day with a relaxing bath; add several drops of lavender oil to help soothe you to sleep. By the next day, your body should be clear of the alcohol residue.

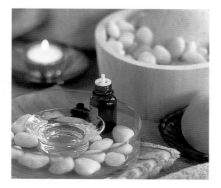

◀ Try not to overtax your system when hungover – relax with some aromatherapy.

73

aromatherapy oils

Aromatic essential oils are used in many ways to promote and restore health, as well as improve the quality of life with their scent. They are extracted from the flowers and foliage of plants and trees.

the oils

SANDALWOOD: A heavy-scented oil with antidepressant properties.

CHAMOMILE: This is a very relaxing, antispasmodic oil that relieves tension headaches and insomnia.

GERANIUM: This rose-scented oil has refreshing, antidepressant properties and is a very good treatment for nervousness and exhaustion.

BENZOIN: Vanilla-scented gum extract from an Asian tree. It is used in inhalation mixtures as it eases restricted breathing.

YLANG YLANG: This pungent oil is from an Indonesian tree and has a sedative, yet antidepressant action. It is good for panic attacks, insomnia, anxiety and depression.

PEPPERMINT: Its strong analgesic and antispasmodic properties make peppermint an ideal treatment for tension headaches.

EUCALYPTUS: One of the best oils for respiratory complaints.

JASMINE: A relaxing, euphoric aroma makes jasmine a great mood lifter.

LAVENDER: Useful for stress-related ailments, burns and skin care, lavender is one of the most versatile oils.

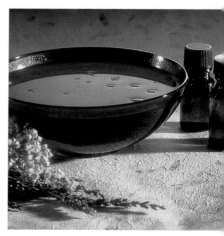

▲ Aromatherapy oils can be dispersed in a bowl of hot water or by using an oil burner.

FENNEL: One of the best detoxifying oils available.

ORANGE: An uplifting and detoxifying oil that helps to combat fluid retention and muscular aches and pains.

CHOOSING OILS
Buy good-quality aromatherapy oils. Blend small amounts at a time, as their healing properties deteriorate when in contact with air. Store in a cool, dark place.

74   aromatherapy massage

A massage with aromatherapy oils is one of the most beneficial ways to ease tension, headaches and stress, and to help release toxins stored in body tissues and cells during a detox programme.

self-massage

Give yourself a break from work or an evening treat by using simple massage techniques. You can concentrate on one section of your body at a time, targetting tired and tense muscles. Choose a blend of essential oils – such as ylang ylang, orange and geranium – and add 1 per cent to a base oil, such as sweet almond or grapeseed oil.

with a partner

Massaging a partner is a great way to share physical contact, and relax and revive each other after a busy working day. Create a warm and comfortable space beforehand, using pillows or cushions for support, and cover his or her body with towels, if needed, to keep warm. Choose an oil blend that you both like, then warm the oil by rubbing it between your hands before applying to the skin.

You may want to light candles, as the diffused light will help you both relax. Calming New Age or classical music will help create a pleasant mood. After one partner has been massaged, you can swap places.

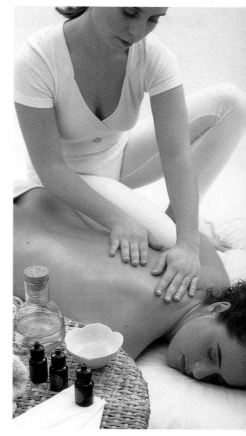

▲ You can practise massage techniques with a partner to boost energy levels.

75 head massage

Massaging the head is a very effective antidote to stress, as it loosens tension in the scalp and benefits the whole body. Keep your hands moving, as one stroke moves into the next.

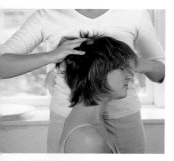

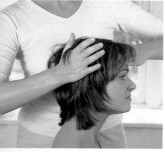

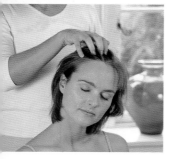

1 Stand to the left of your partner and support their forehead with your left hand. Put your right hand at the front of their face before the ear by the hairline. Using three or four fingers, rub the scalp briskly back and forth in a vigorous sawing movement.

2 Without stopping, use the heel of your right hand to rub briskly over the whole head. Use firmer pressure at the base of the skull. Repeat three times.

3 Standing behind your partner, slide both your hands round to the side of the head. Spread your fingers wide and, with slow, deliberate movements, make small circles, applying pressure with your fingertips. You should feel their scalp moving slightly. Work across the whole head. Repeat three times.

4 Starting at the top of the forehead at the hairline, rake your fingers backwards through the hair. Use both hands one after the other to make the stroke continuous. Work over the whole head three times. Repeat this action three times with a slower, gentle ruffling movement.

5 Starting at the front of the hairline, use the whole of your hand to lightly stroke over your partner's head. Let one hand follow the other in a continuous movement and work down to the base of the skull. Work over the whole head a number of times.

76 hand massage

For people who use computers, machinists and musicians, the hands may easily become strained through extended use. Regular breaks and self-massage can prevent repetitive strain injury.

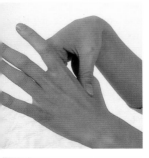

1 To release stored tensions and improve circulation, start by squeezing between each finger in turn, with the thumb and index finger of the other hand.

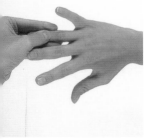

2 Make a rolling movement on each finger, slowly working your way from the knuckle to the fingertip, with firm pressure.

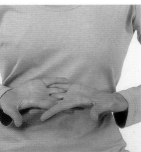

3 Stretch each digit with a gentle pulling action to ease tight tendons – there is no need to "crack" each finger. Interlock the fingers of both hands and stretch the palms.

4 Finally, make a circling motion with one thumb on the palm of the other hand. This squeezes and stretches taut, contracted muscles. It should be a fairly deep action. Work all over the palm, maintaining a firm and even pressure.

EQUAL SIDES
Once you have completed steps 1 to 4, repeat each massage technique on the opposite hand.

self-massage

You can choose a relevant stroke from this self-massage sequence or do it all. Repeat each stroke using the other hand. Make sure you are sitting comfortably with enough spinal support.

1 Place your working hand on the opposite shoulder. Cup your other hand over the elbow and push your working hand as far down the upper back as is comfortable. Using the pads of your fingers make circular strokes, working upwards over the muscles between the shoulder blade and the spine. Repeat twice more.

2 Place your working hand near the base of your neck on the opposite shoulder. Gently squeeze the muscle that starts here and work your way along the top of the shoulder, down the upper arm to the elbow. Increase the pressure as you go if comfortable. Hold and release. Repeat three times.

3 With your working hand at the base of the neck on the opposite shoulder, dig your fingertips into the muscles. Using a circular action, work along the tops and backs of the shoulder muscles. Work from the base of the neck out to the end of the shoulder. Repeat three times.

4 Place the thumb of your working hand in the hollow behind the collarbone. Using your other fingers pinch and release along the top of the shoulder; this might be painful if your muscles are tight, so breathe out as you pinch. This stroke is very effective for releasing muscles that are taut or in spasm.

5 Place one hand on your forehead and your working hand at the back of the neck. Tilt your head forwards a little. Starting at the top of the neck, use circular finger strokes to roll down the sides of the neck. Then use your whole hand to squeeze and pull down the back of the neck. Repeat three times.

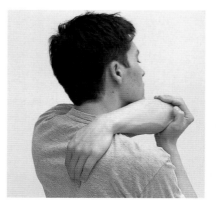

78

five-minute fix

When you don't have time for a complete self-massage sequence, this five-minute routine will give you a boost. Based on shiatsu-style massage it works on your energy channels.

1 Sit with your shoes off. Spread out your toes and plant your feet firmly on the ground. Cup your left elbow in the palm of your right hand and use your left knuckles to tap the right side of the body. Tap down the side of the neck and continue over the top of the shoulder and down into the upper back. Work as far down the back as you can, using your hand on your elbow for leverage. Repeat on the other side.

2 Continue tapping down the outside of your arm to your hand (*see right*). Then tap on the inside all the way up to the armpit, over the shoulder joint and then back down the outside of the arm once more. Repeat three times, then swap hands and do the other arm.

3 Now use the same tapping stroke on your chest. Sit back in the chair and, keeping your wrists soft, tap across the upper chest. Work from the middle of your chest outwards towards the shoulder. This is a very invigorating and sometimes quite amusing movement. Repeat three times.

4 Place your feet slightly apart on the ground, and pummel down the outside of both legs at the same time. Repeat this action three times. Finish by pummelling up the inside of both legs. Repeat three times. Slowly sit up and take a deep breath to finish.

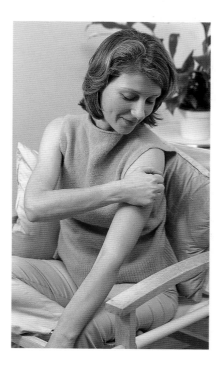

79 stomach & chest massage

Emotional tension is often stored in the torso – these bottled-up feelings may cause tight muscles across the chest and abdomen. Self-massage can help you release the stress.

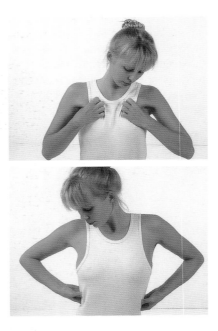

1 Using thumbs and fingers, grip your pectoral muscles on both sides of the chest leading towards the shoulders. Knead them firmly. If you have any tenderness in the breasts and lymph glands beneath the armpits (ie, women who are premenstrual), use a more gentle pressure.

2 With a couple of fingers, feel in between the ribs for the intercostal muscles. Work firmly between each rib, moving the fingers in tiny circles. Repeat on each side.

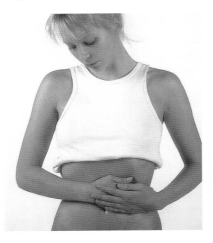

3 Place your hands on your abdomen, and apply pressure slowly in a clockwise direction. Repeat a couple of times with increasing pressure, but ease off if this becomes painful – it is best not to overdo it. This action promotes digestive and bowel action.

80

buttocks & thigh massage

For people whose jobs involve being on their feet all day, the thighs and buttocks can take a beating. This set of massage exercises will benefit aching muscles and restore circulation in swollen limbs.

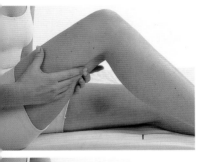

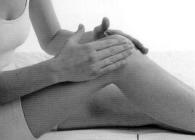

1 Start by working up the sides of the thighs. Using both hands, knead one thigh at a time, applying a firm pressure by squeezing muscles between the fingers and thumb.

2 Squeeze with each hand alternatively for the best effect, working from the front of the knee to the hip and back. Repeat on the other thigh.

3 Rising to a kneeling position, pummel your hips and buttocks, using a clenched fist and keeping your wrists flexible. This will get your circulation moving and also help to loosen cellulite in the tissues.

UPLIFTING OILS
Citrus oils have a tonic effect on the limbs; try adding a few drops of orange and lemon oil to a hot bath after your massage.

81 leg massage

Calves and knees may ache following physical exertion such as hiking, tennis, dancing and step and aerobic exercises. This massage sequence will allow your limbs to return to a neutral state.

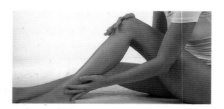

1 Sit in a comfortable position with one leg bent, so that you can easily reach down as far as your ankle.

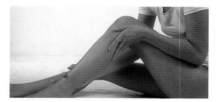

2 Stroke the leg lightly with both hands from ankle to thigh, repeating several times. Move the leg slightly each time to reach a different part. This will have a warming effect on the limbs.

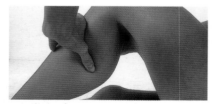

3 Using steady, firm pressure, work up the leg from ankle to knee with a squeezing action, paying particular attention to the back of the calves. This helps to move venous blood back towards the heart, and ease tension.

4 Massage the knee, slowly stroking around the outside of the kneecap, then use a circular pressure to move around the kneecaps more firmly with the fingertips.

82 swiss reflex therapy

Areas of the body have reflexes located in the feet, and massaging these can have a therapeutic effect. Pressure on a blocked reflex can be painful, so work to your own pain threshold for one minute.

3 For a long area like the spine, do a small area at a time, moving down and repeating until all the spine (inside edge of the foot) has been covered. Change your hand position, depending on the reflex being treated. You may need to consult a reflexology chart to locate problem areas.

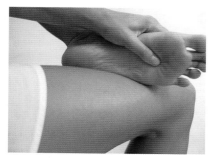

1 Start any reflex therapy by working just below the ball of the foot (the solar plexus reflex area) in order to relax the body. Rest your right foot on the knee of your left leg and massage with the whole length of your right thumb in a circular motion. Keep circling, maintaining the same pressure, until the discomfort has completely gone. If after a minute it is painful, the original pressure may have been too strong.

2 Using a circular movement again, massage any reflex areas that present a problem. For example, the lung reflex area (which is in the centre of the ball of the foot) if you have bronchial problems, and the spinal areas (the entire inside edge of each foot) for backache, muscle pains, rheumatism or arthritis.

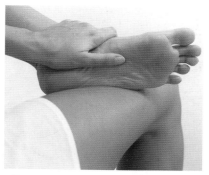

4 Finish by massaging the full length of your right thumb in a firm oval movement, over the kidney-urethra-bladder (under the highest point of the foot arch) area to help eliminate any released toxins. Apply the pressure from kidney to bladder area, with no pressure being applied on the return half of the circle. Repeat the sequence on your left foot, changing hands.

83 aerobic exercise

Aerobic exercises are those that raise the heart rate. Sustained by oxygen, they burn fat, boost the immune system and exercise the heart. Include them in detox to increase stamina and flexibility.

how to exercise

Walking, jogging, cycling and swimming all offer excellent aerobic exercise – with the bonus being that they are inexpensive and fun. Most gyms offer aerobics classes that use steps or weights, and these may be high or low impact. Choose a class that matches your fitness level. Dancing is another enjoyable way to exercise; many gyms offer classes in salsa, samba and ceroc, for example.

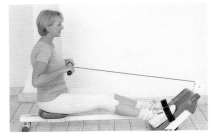

▲ Use simple exercise devices to get your aerobic activity during bad weather.

detox benefits

When following a detox plan, aerobics will help accelerate weight loss and eliminate toxins from the system. But go gently – you will not be consuming your usual amount of "fuel" in calories, so if you feel faint or light–headed, stop immediately. Remember to drink plenty of water.

stay motivated

Make exercise part of your daily routine by walking to work or on short journeys, such as collecting the children from school.

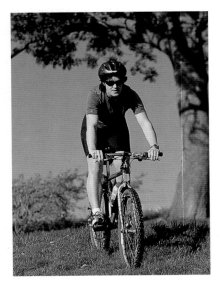

◄ If you choose to exercise alone, cycling is a good way to get outdoors.

84 anaerobic exercise

Anaerobic exercise is a way of improving muscle strength and flexibility without vigorous exertion. It burns plenty of carbohydrates and can also boost your metabolism to burn fat indirectly.

low-impact exercise

There are three types of anaerobic, or "low-impact" exercise:
- isotonics – muscles contract against a resistant object
- isometrics – muscles contract against a resistant object without movement to build strength without bulk
- calisthenics – stretching exercises to increase flexibility and joint mobility.

a regular routine

The types of exercise you choose will depend on what you enjoy as much as your physical ability, but a good programme will include anaerobic as well as aerobic exercise. Joining a gym will get you professional advice, but you can follow a routine at home.

Be sure to include warming up and winding down exercises. Work slowly and evenly and with some tension in your limbs, as if they are resisting a weight. If you are new to a routine, stop if you feel pain.

▼ Alternate running and walking to build endurance and strength.

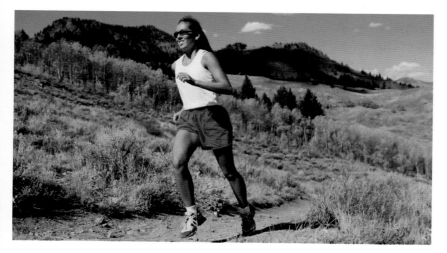

85 breathing

We breathe without thought for the effort the action takes, 24 hours and day, 7 days a week. Yet focusing on our breathing and learning to breathe more deeply can have positive benefits for us.

deep breathing

Practising these exercises during detox will give you greater control over your breathing and help you to centre your thoughts, allowing you to focus on your goals. You can use them at work, at home or any time to invoke a feeling of peacefulness.

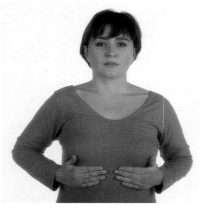

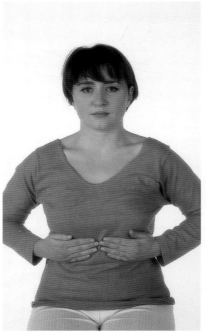

1 Place your hands just below the breastbone and take slow, deep breaths. As you breathe in, push out your stomach. This should make your hands move apart a little, and indicates that the diaphragm is moving as it should.

2 As you gently breathe out, slowly pull in your stomach muscles. Your diaphragm will move back upwards, and your hands will come together again. Repeat this exercise three or four times, and then begin to breathe normally again.

86 calming the mind

With so many activities, cares and responsibilities packed into a day, it is easy to feel overwhelmed. Meditation helps calm the mind, enabling you to approach tasks feeling balanced and refreshed.

prepare to meditate

Set aside a quiet place, perhaps lighting a candle or burning incense. You can sit cross-legged on a cushion, or recline on a bed or sofa. The following meditation can be recorded on tape if you find it helpful to listen to the sound of the words.

the haven

In this meditation, you will find your own special place – real or imaginary – in which to rest and feel safe. Close your eyes and allow your mind to drift. Where is this special place?

It may be a place you visited as a child, in a quiet corner of a wood or a secret room in a ruined castle, where you found yourself suddenly away from other people. Go to the place ... feel what made it special ... what makes it special still ... it belongs only to you, so you can think and do whatever you like ...

Notice what sort of light shines in through the branches outside the window ... is it bright or hazy? ... Does the temperature feel soothingly warm or refreshingly cool? ... Be aware of the colours that surround

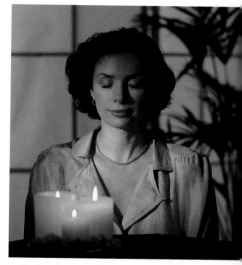

▲ During detox, meditation helps cleanse the mind of debris, as well as the body.

you ... the outlines of shapes ... the textures ... What sounds do you hear? ... Distant voices, church bells or perhaps birds singing ...

No one is asking anything of you ... no one expects anything of you ... you don't need to be anywhere ... except here, a place where everything is peaceful and you can truly relax and let yourself go ...

visualization

Simple visualization techniques can help you cope with stress. By letting your imagination "see" beyond the current crisis, you can register new ideas and ways of dealing with difficult people and situations.

the protective bubble

Imagine that you are in a situation that has, in the past, made you feel anxious. Picture the location and the people involved. See yourself there with them ... and notice a slight shimmer of light surrounding you, a sort of glowing "bubble" between you and the other people ... a protective bubble that reflects any negative feelings back on to them,

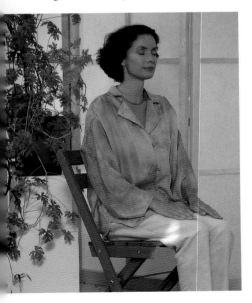

leaving you the space to get on with your work, your life and developing your inner strength and calmness.

Concentrate on the bubble that surrounds and protects you at all times. It will only allow positive feelings to pass through, for you to enjoy and build upon. Others may feel negativity, but you are protected ... you can deal with whatever comes across your path in a calm and clear way. You are able to see the way forward ... solve problems ... find your way around difficulties ... by using your own rich inner resources and talents.

Imagine pushing out through the bubble emotions that are unhelpful ... such as jealousy, embarrassments, past resentments ... Push them out to where they can no longer harm or hinder you. Now you can keep things in better perspective, accepting the things you cannot change. You can control the way you think and act ... how you deal with others ... and move on with confidence and happiness.

◀ *Visualizations to improve your overall confidence levels can act as a rehearsal for future situations.*

88 stretches

When the limbs become tired, through tension or fatigue, the contraction of the muscles can lead to poor circulation. A few simple stretches can help restore the blood supply and relieve tight muscles.

blood flow enhancer

Chronic stress can make you feel tight across the chest and make your hands feel cold. This exercise will facilitate blood flow, allowing you to breathe more deeply, which will nourish all the cells in the body and warm the extremities.

STRETCHING EXERCISES
Practise simple stretching exercises during detox to help release toxins from the tissues.

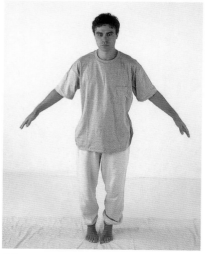

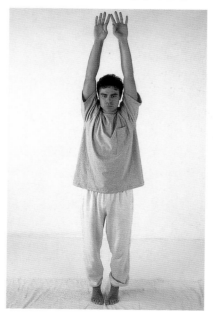

1 Stand with your feet close together and your arms resting by your sides. Slowly take a deep breath in, and at the same time, raise your arms out to your sides. Rise up on your toes.

2 Raise your arms until they meet directly over your head. As you exhale, slowly return to the original position. Repeat the sequence just three or four times more.

A German–style sitz bath enables buttocks and hips to be immersed in hot water as a soothing therapy after certain types of surgery

90 salt bath

A bath with Epsom salts will help to eliminate toxins from the skin by drawing out impurities, leaving your body feeling wonderfully smooth and firm. Use during the 7-day detox.

taking a salt bath

As you run warm water into the bath, pour 450g/1lb of Epsom salts under the tap, so that they dissolve and disperse. Lie back in a comfortable position for 20 minutes, adding more hot water if the bath becomes too cool.

Afterwards, pat your skin dry, wrap yourself up in a warm towel and relax for an hour, or go to bed. You may sweat during the night, so drink plenty of water before you go to sleep and plenty in the morning. When you wake, take a normal bath or shower to remove any salty residues.

CAUTION

- If you suffer from high blood pressure, it is best to avoid the Epsom salts bath.

▾ Epsom salts are very high in magnesium, a soothing balm for tired, aching muscles.

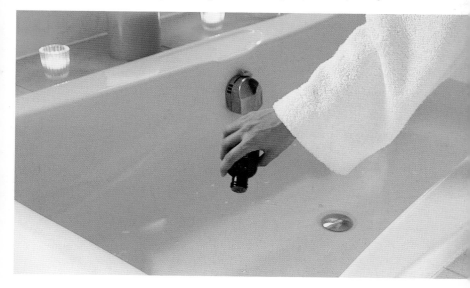

91

body scrub

Although fairly new in the West, body scrubs have been a Middle Eastern tradition for centuries. Use a body scrub whenever you feel the need for a deep cleanse that will promote good circulation.

citrus body scrub

The slightly gritty texture of this freshly scented exfoliating scrub helps to remove dead skin cells and stimulates the blood supply, leaving your skin feeling tingling and well toned. The recipe makes enough for five treatments.

45ml/3 tbsp ground sunflower seeds
45ml/3 tbsp medium oatmeal
45ml/3 tbsp flaked sea salt
45ml/3 tbsp grated orange peel
15ml/1 tbsp grated lemon peel
3 drops grapefruit essential oil
glass jar with lid
almond oil

Mix all the ingredients thoroughly and store in the sealed glass jar. When ready for a treatment, make a paste with ⅕ of the scrub and some almond oil in a shallow bowl. Remove all your clothes and stand in the bath. Gently massage the scrub all over your body, paying particular attention to areas of hard, dry skin such as the elbows, knees and ankles. Remove the residue before showering or bathing.

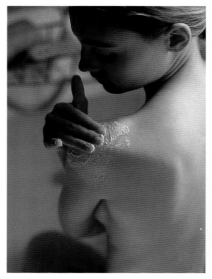

▲ An exfoliating body scrub will leave your skin glowing and healthy.

WHEN TO USE
• Use a body scrub before moisturizing your skin and before applying tanning lotion.

• Body scrubs are a perfect way to perk up winter skin during dark, cold months when it does not receive much sunshine.

92   skin brushing

Brushing the skin with a dry, natural bristle brush is an exhilarating way to boost your circulation. Not only does it make your skin feel smooth, it stimulates the senses and helps to eliminate cellulite.

10-minute routine

The whole process of skin brushing should take about 10 minutes – this is plenty of time to go over your entire body. Try brushing in the morning before taking a bath or shower. Skin brushing will also help the effectiveness of an aromatherapy bath, making your skin and pores more open to the oils.

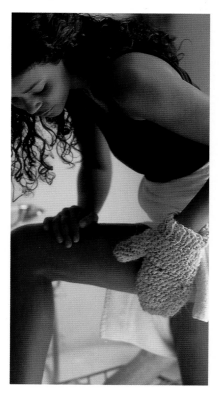

> **HOW TO BRUSH SKIN**
>
> 1 Start with your feet and toes. Using long strokes (towards your heart), brush up the front and back of your legs. Move up to your thighs and groin area.
>
> 2 Brush over your buttocks, up to the lower back.
>
> 3 Now brush gently along your hands and arms, inwards towards the heart.
>
> 4 Gently brush your stomach, using circular, clockwise motions.
>
> 5 Move across your shoulders, down over your chest (lightly over the breasts). Finally, move down your back, towards your heart.

▸ *For super-soft skin, brush gently with a sisal mitt or brush in the bath or shower.*

93 saunas & steam baths

Traditionally, hot dry or steam baths have been utilized by many peoples, from Scandinavians to Native Americans. They have the power to purify body, mind and soul.

a detox bath

Saunas and steam baths work by encouraging perspiration (sweat) and boosting the circulation, which in turn help eliminate toxins from the system. It is best to spend between 5–10 minutes in the heat at a time, then take a cold shower or swim in between. Finish your session with a cold shower, then relax for 30 minutes until your body has adjusted to its normal temperature.

CAUTION
- If you suffer from heart problems or high blood pressure, avoid saunas and steam baths.

- It is a good idea to abstain from eating heavy meals, or drinking alcohol and caffeine before taking a sauna or steam bath.

▾ *You can use the time after a cleansing sauna or steam bath to relax and meditate.*

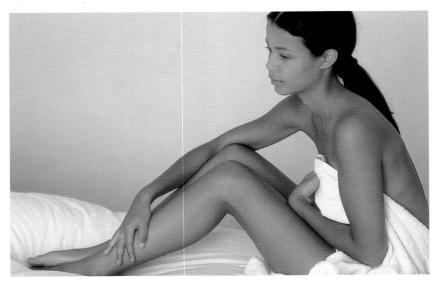

94 mud wrap

The healing properties of mud are well known around the world. When used as a skin wrap, its high mineral content nourishes the body, heals wounds, clears rashes and reduces cellulite.

spa treatment

The best way to get a full mud wrap is to pamper yourself and visit one of the many spas that offer the treatment. A special mud – which may also contain herbs and spices – is smeared all over your body; following this, you are wrapped in a plastic sheet. Towels are wrapped around you to keep your body temperature even while the mud works to draw out impurities. After perspiring gently for about 20 minutes, you can take a shower, pat yourself dry and then luxuriate in the smooth and clean texture of your skin.

types of mud

Mud wraps use various types of local mud, each of which has its own special properties. White Thai mud, also called *din so porng*, is mixed with turmeric, marjoram and spring water – it has antiperspirant, coolant and moisturizing properties. In Northern California, a local mud mixed with crushed Napa Valley grape seeds purifies and tones the skin, while Moor mud, which is rich in black magma, minerals, amino antibodies

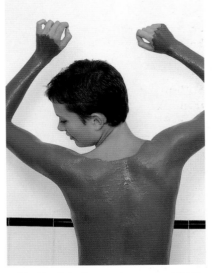

▲ *Ideal for detoxing, mud wraps work from the outside-in to promote good health.*

and salicylic acid (the substance used in aspirin) relieves rheumatic aches and injuries.

> **GLORIOUS MUD**
> Mud face masks promote a glowing complexion and are easy to use at home.

95 face scrub

The face is subject to the ill effects of weather, pollution and often alcohol and cigarette smoke. Exfoliating delicate tissues with a gentle face scrub will leave your skin feeling soft and renewed.

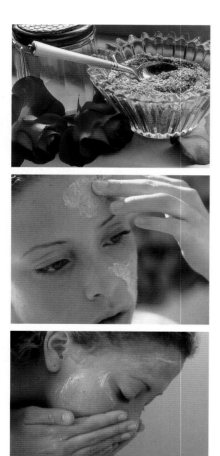

Treat yourself to the following all-natural, rose-scented face scrub. It is best to choose pure, organic ingredients; these will be readily available from many supermarkets and health food stores. You can purchase the rose petals from a herbalist – or pick, dry and powder blooms from your own garden. This recipe makes enough for about ten treatments.

cleopatra face scrub
45ml/3 tbsp ground almonds
45ml/3 tbsp medium oatmeal
45ml/3 tbsp powdered milk
30ml/2 tbsp powdered rose petals
glass jar with lid
almond oil

Mix all the dry ingredients together in the jar. Before using, mix a small portion with almond oil to form a soft paste. With the lightest touch, rub the mixture into your skin, using a gentle circular motion. Be careful to avoid the delicate area around your eyes. Finally, rinse off the face scrub with warm water and pat your face dry with a soft towel.

96 steam facial

Steam facials open the pores and deep-clean the skin: the heat relaxes the pores and boosts blood circulation. With the addition of herbs and flowers, the stimulating and cleansing action is magnified.

rose and chamomile facial

Fill a bowl just wider than your face with hot water, and add 3 drops of rose essential oil and 4 drops of chamomile essential oil. Cover your head with a towel, draping it over the bowl. Let steam waft over your face for 5 minutes, then relax in a quiet place for a further 15 minutes before closing the pores.

Dab cooled skin with one of the following toners: for dry skin, mix 75ml/5 tbsp triple-distilled rose water with 30ml/2 tbsp orange flower water. Oily skins should use 90ml/6 tbsp rose water mixed with 30ml/2 tbsp witch hazel. Store concoctions in clean bottles and keep cool or refrigerate.

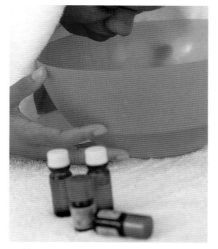

▲ After an aromatherapy facial, you will be confident that your skin looks its best.

fresh facials

Instead of using essential oils, float fresh flowers and leaves, such as chamomile or rose petals, in hot water. You could also try mint, marjoram, lavender or marigold.

> **CAUTION**
> Do not use a steam facial if you are prone to thread veins.

▼ The power of a flower's scent leaves you feeling refreshed and rejuvenated.

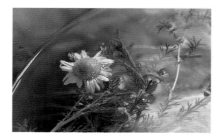

mouth cleansing

The mouth is an area where cleanliness is particularly important. Many herbs can be used to keep the breath fresh and the teeth white – you can make your own natural mixtures for oral hygiene.

mouthwashes and tooth powder

Home-made herbal preparations are far gentler than commercial antiseptic mouthwashes, which can upset the natural acid balance of the mouth. To use one of these pleasant-tasting mouthwashes, swish the liquid around inside the mouth for 30 seconds then spit it out.

You can also use a home-mixed herb and salt powder as a natural alternative to toothpaste. Use it sprinkled on a damp toothbrush.

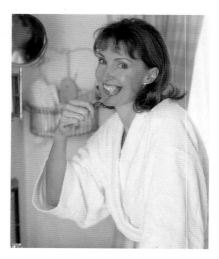

spicy lemon verbena mouthwash

5ml/1 tsp each ground nutmeg, ground cloves, cardamom pods and caraway seeds
small handful fresh lemon verbena leaves or 15g/½ oz dried verbena
600ml/1 pint/2½ cups purified water
30ml/2 tbsp sweet sherry

Place the spices and the lemon verbena leaves in a pan. Pour in the water and simmer for 30 minutes. Strain through a sieve and discard the spices and verbena. Add the sherry and pour into a clean bottle.

To use this mouthwash, dilute 15-30ml/1-2 tbsp in a glass of water.

lavender mouthwash

15ml/1 tbsp dried lavender
300ml/½ pint/1¼ cups purified water
30ml/2 tbsp sweet sherry

Simmer the lavender in the water for 30 minutes. Strain, add the sherry and pour into a clean bottle. Use diluted as for verbena mouthwash.

◄ *A glowing smile and fresh breath are not only attractive, they signal good health.*

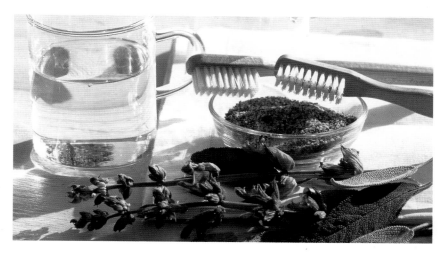

sage-and-salt tooth powder
25g/1oz fresh sage leaves
60ml/4 tbsp sea salt

With a pair of scissors, shred the sage leaves finely and scatter them into an ovenproof dish. Grind the sea salt into the leaves with a wooden spoon or pestle. Bake the ground mixture at 140°C/275°F/Gas 1 for about 1 hour, until the sage is dry and crisp. Pound it down again until it is reduced to a fine powder.

SIMPLE BREATH FRESHENERS
- Chew the fresh-picked leaves of parsley, watercress or mint after eating a meal with garlic or onions.
- Suck or chew on fennel and caraway seeds, star anise, angelica or cloves.
- Dilute half-and-half rose water with mineral water and use the mixture as a mouthrinse.

gargles
For sore throats, voice loss and colds that may go to the chest, gargling with one or more essential oils can be very helpful. Put 2–3 drops of antibacterial essential oils into a glass and half-fill with water. Alternatively infuse sage and thyme leaves in boiling water. Stir well, take a mouthful, gargle and spit out. Stir again and repeat. It is important to stir the mixture before each mouthful so as to redisperse the oils. For the best results, gargle twice a day.

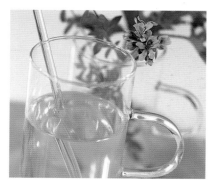

98 hair detox

Many people wash, condition and style too often, resulting in a build-up of commercial products that contain chemicals and additives. Give your hair a detox treat by making your own herbal hair rinses.

Make up one of these fresh rinses in a jug before you begin washing. Hold your head over a bowl as you pour the herbal rinse through your hair, then pour back the rinse from the bowl to the jug. Reapply at least five times for really shiny hair.

rosemary rinse for dark hair
40g/1½ oz fresh rosemary sprigs
1 litre/1¾ pints/4 cups boiling water

Put the sprigs in a jug and pour in the boiling water. Leave to stand and steep for 1 hour, then strain off the herbs through a sieve. Because of the high essential oil content of rosemary, the rinse is also good for dry hair.

chamomile rinse for fair hair
25g/1oz dried chamomile flowers or 40g/1½oz fresh flowers and leaves
1 litre/1¾pints/4 cups boiling water

Prepare and use this rinse in the same way as the dark hair rosemary rinse described above.

▸ *Natural hair rinses are inexpensive and will keep your locks healthy and shiny.*

nettle rinse for dandruff
1 litre/1¾ pints/4 cups boiling water
25g/1oz fresh nettle leaves
25g/1oz nasturtium flowers
30ml/2 tbsp cider vinegar
30ml/2 tbsp witch hazel

Pour the water over the nettles and nasturtiums (nettles lose their sting in boiling water). Leave to stand overnight, then strain off the herbs, and add vinegar and witch hazel. Pour through as a final rinse every time you shampoo.

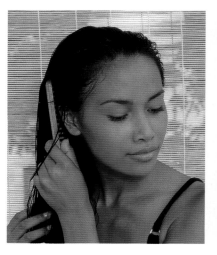

enriching oil treatments

Instead of using a manufactured hair conditioner, for a change why not try a pre-wash Indian oil massage? It's an intense treatment that stimulates the scalp as well as coating the hair shaft. The series of movements aims to stimulate the body's nervous systems, including glands, nerves and circulation, with anti-aging effects.

Apply the oil using vigorous circular motions of the palms and fingertips to work it well into the scalp and down the length of the hair. After the massage, wrap a towel round your head, and leave it on for a few hours or overnight. You may need to vary the amount of shampoo you use.

warming and cooling oils

Oil is used to strengthen and nourish all kinds of hair, but the treatment should be tailored to suit the person. Your choice of oil should also be influenced by external conditions such as the weather or time of the year. Coconut oil is popular for head massage, as it is renowned for its nourishing and strengthening properties. But it also has a cooling effect, which means it's best used in hot weather.

In the winter, use a warming oil such as mustard or olive. Mustard is very nourishing and has a strong heating effect, though it smells rather strong. Almond is more neutral and has a slightly warming effect.

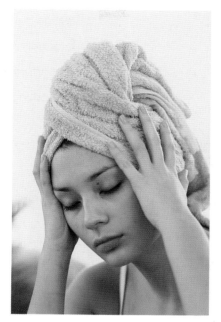

▲ *If you don't want to leave oil on your hair for long, wrap your head in a warm, damp towel after applying it, in order to aid penetration.*

warmth and penetration

Warming the oil before you use it on your hair can help it penetrate the hair shaft more effectively. Heat it very slightly in a non-metallic bowl over a pan of water. It should be no more than comfortably warm. Alternatively, wring out a towel in hot water and wrap it around your head when you have applied the oil and again after massaging it in. Again, you need to ensure that the heat is not uncomfortable.

99 foot soaks

Soaking the feet in a hot, invigorating bath not only thoroughly refreshes your feet, but it can lift your mood as well: the warmth relaxes your body and the soothing herbs calm your mind.

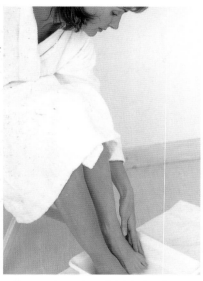

▲ Foot soaks are beneficial during detox – they also soothe colds, flu or chills.

mustard foot bath
15ml/1 tbsp mustard powder
2.2 litres/4 pints/9 cups hot water

Stir the mustard into the water until it is dissolved. Immerse the feet while the bath is still hot. Reheat if required.

▸ A foot bath revitalizes the whole body.

herb foot bath for aching feet
50g/2oz mixed fresh herbs:
    peppermint, yarrow, pine needles,
    chamomile flowers, rosemary
1 litre/1¾ pints/4 cups boiling water
1.75 litres/3 pints/7½ cups hot water
15ml/1 tbsp borax
15ml/1 tbsp Epsom salts

Roughly chop the herbs, place into a large bowl and pour in the boiling water. Leave to stand for 1 hour. Strain, and add to a basin containing the hot water; the final temperature of the foot bath should be comfortably warm. Stir in the borax and Epsom salts, immerse your feet and soak for 15–20 minutes.

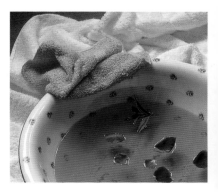

For a tropical treat, pick magnolia, jasmine, hibiscus and rose blossoms, and stew in a hot bath. Lie back and luxuriate in the heady scent.

eternal you

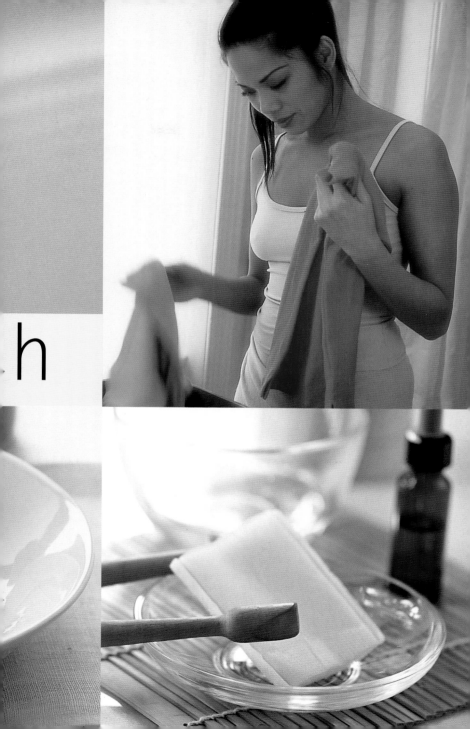

h

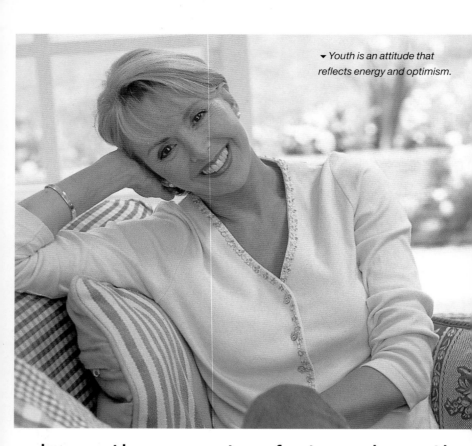

Youth is an attitude that reflects energy and optimism.

learn the secrets of eternal youth

As the population of the developed world enjoys an ever-increasing life span, more and more people are starting to reassess their approach to living and growing older. But growing older doesn't have to follow the traditional definition of aging – "aging" is what happens when we adopt destructive health habits and pessimistic mind sets.

It is possible to enjoy being forty, fifty or eighty years old and still be youthful; it all comes down to your attitude – and how well you take care of yourself. There are ways of staying younger than your chronological age, and many people achieve this by watching what they eat and how they exercise, sleep, relate to other people and deal with life's challenges. When you stop and consider that the wisdom you have gleaned from experience can benefit others, it makes sense to care for yourself, body and soul, to make the most of what you can offer the world.

water power

Probably the most essential ingredient for running the body's systems at optimal levels is water. Playing a major part in digesting foods and absorbing nutrients, water must be replenished almost constantly for the body to stay young and healthy – it is the one thing we cannot live without for very long.

The average person living in a temperate climate needs around eight large glasses of water a day – more in hotter climates or when exercising. Tea and coffee do not count in this quota. Drinking this amount will not only help keep your weight down, it will flush toxins out of the system, leaving your skin glowing – and beautiful skin is the most obvious indicator of youth and vigour.

food and exercise

Research into longevity has shown that by slowly reducing calories consumed over a period of years, the human life span can be prolonged. A diet high in fruit, vegetables and fibre and low in saturated fats is also beneficial. This doesn't mean that you can never enjoy high-calorie treats – only that it is best to modify your eating habits and keep an eye on sound nutrition most of the time.

Exercise works not only to boost the metabolism, so that the body responds from a younger fitness level, it also lifts the spirits, helping to energize and enthuse the mind, and keep depression at bay.

▼ *Replace your tea and coffee intake with refreshing herbal teas.*

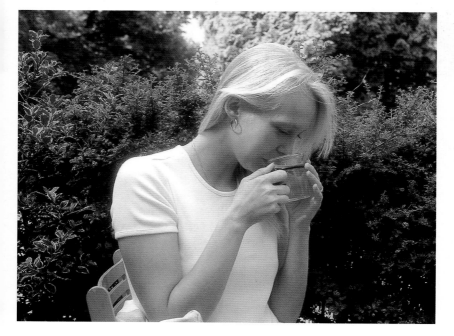

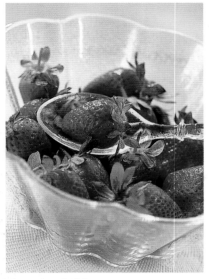

term heavy smoker. Their skin is sallow, teeth and lips yellow, and they may cough and get short of breath running up stairs. Kicking the habit is the best way to prevent lung disease.

supplemental help

As more research into aging is carried out, new information on beneficial substances comes to light. Many can be manufactured by the body, but the modern diet does not provide the necessary nutrients. Also, larger quantities of substances such as glucosamine sulphate – derived from seashells, which we do not normally eat – can be beneficial, in this case, protecting joints and cartilage. The antioxidant effects of tea polyphenols, grapeseed extract and co-enzyme Q-10 can work rejuvenating wonders.

soul food

Knowing when to ask for help is an important part of living in a society. No one is perfect or omnipotent, and sharing your problems – and joys – with family, friends and partners is helpful both for you and for them; giving is as important as receiving. Likewise, developing a sense of your own identity – exploring your feelings, thoughts and creativity – is crucial for wellbeing. Seeing yourself as a spiritual entity in the grand scheme of things puts your place in the world into perspective, and provides a good vantage point for a long and happy life.

changing habits

There is no doubt that avoiding eating certain foods, moderating your alcohol intake and giving up smoking are just as important as good nutrition and proper sleep. Reducing your fat and sugar intake is essential, as excesses overload the system, leading to imbalances and diseases such as diabetes and heart conditions. It is a good idea to cut out processed foods too – heating destroys crucial enzymes, and chemicals are often added.

Alcohol can play havoc with the system, especially as you grow older – drinking places stress on the liver, impairs the uptake of nutrients and damages cells. Cigarette smoking is one of the most destructive things you can do to your body, and one of the quickest ways to accelerate aging. You may think that it helps you to stay thin, or increases enjoyment of social activity – but take one look at a long-

Close relationships will keep you feeling youthful and happy.

anti-aging
treatments

This chapter outlines fundamental ways in which you can help stay the aging process. Sections on low-calorie and raw-fruit diets describe the foundations of nutritious eating, and information on choosing proteins, healthy fats, fibre and minerals completes the overall picture.

Supplements – from important antioxidants to brain-boosting herbs such as gingko biloba – can give your health and appearance a real boost. Calcium helps stave off osteoporosis, and B vitamins rejuvenate both mind and body.

Exercise is just as important as diet: included is information on aerobics and anaerobics, yoga and Tai Chi. Learning to deal effectively with stress and depression is a key to longevity, as are positive thinking, getting enough sleep and treating yourself to rejuvenating therapies.

Finally, enjoy the company of other people, have fun and develop a strong sense of your own identity and spirituality to be sure of the lengthiest and most fulfilled of lives.

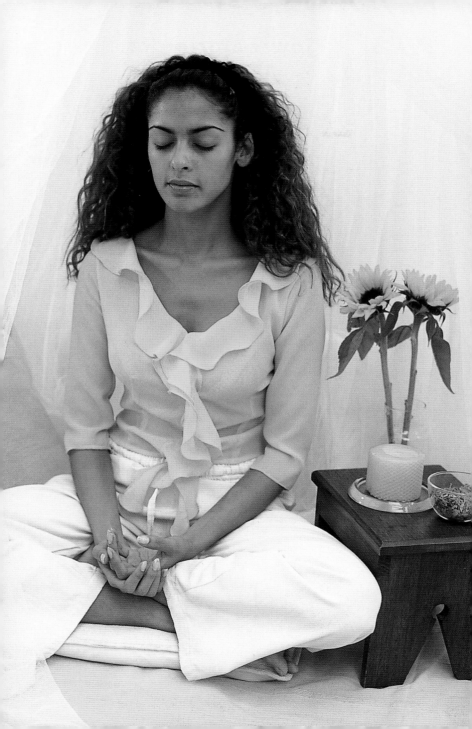

101 low-calorie diet

Research into longevity has shown that by reducing the total number of calories consumed daily, you can effectively prolong life – retaining health and youthful looks in the process.

Overeating is one of the worst age accelerators – it places stress on all of the body's systems, as digestion burns up extra energy that could be used for other functions. In addition, excess food causes weight gain, and excess fat is implicated in many age-onset diseases, such as heart disease and diabetes. This all boils down to one simple conclusion: if you eat less, you will live longer.

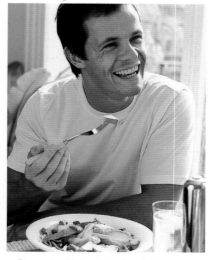

▲ Swapping high-calorie foods for more raw foods such as salads may extend your life.

important biomarkers

Biomarkers are factors that indicate how much younger you are physiologically than your chronological age. They include skin dryness, greying hair and blood cholesterol. Research with laboratory animals found great improvements when the animals were put on reduced-calorie diets; they lived longer, healthier lives than those who ate what they wanted.

slow decrease

Eating less does not mean skimping on nutrition – it means replacing high-calorie foods containing excess fats and sugars with raw, nutritious foods. It is suggested that, starting in middle age, the anti-aging diet should involve decreasing the amount of calories consumed to 60% of what you would normally eat – gradually, over a period of five to seven years.

This means reducing calories to 1,800 for men and 1,300 for women; slightly more for very active people. This controlled undernutrition effectively lowers body temperature and decreases metabolic rate, two major factors in increased longevity.

102 raw power

Following a diet high in raw foods – particularly fruit – is an achievable way to help you stay young. The enzymes in fresh, "live" foods act to keep the body's systems working at premium levels.

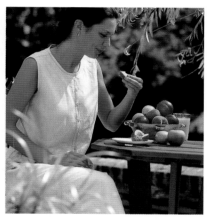

▲ *Eat fresh fruits slowly, chewing many times to release beneficial enzymes.*

When food is cooked, important enzymes are destroyed, so eating it raw, or juicing it for drinking immediately, ensures optimum levels of nutrients. Evidence suggests that a diet made up of 50% raw fruit can lengthen the life span. In fact, age researchers claim that a diet with 70% raw fruit and vegetables may actually begin to reverse the aging process: the body becomes leaner; wrinkles appear smoother and all-important brain function improves considerably.

TOP FRUITS

Although all fruits are good, some are particularly potent anti-agers. Choose organic fruits where possible, as they are free from pesticides – and they taste better.

- **Apples** Excellent detoxifiers with antiseptic qualities, which strengthen the immune system. Apples also contain pectin, which binds heavy metals such as lead and mercury and carries them out of the body.
- **Kiwi fruit** Containing double the vitamin C of oranges, twice as much vitamin E as an avocado, and a rich store of potassium, kiwis are wonderful.
- **Berries** Blackberries, blueberries, blackcurrants and black grapes contain phytochemicals known as flavonoids, potent antioxidants that protect against damage caused by free radicals.
- **Lemons** Very effective at flushing toxins from the system.
- **Dates and figs** Rich in calcium, iron and potassium, these are also good for digestion.

103 vital vegetables

Providing minerals, bioflavonoids, antioxidants, phytochemicals and protein, vegetables are essential for rejuvenating cell growth – and they make a delicious, colourful feast.

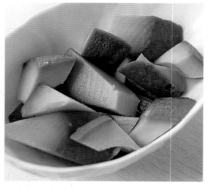

▲ Avocado is an excellent source of skin-enhancing vitamin E and unsaturated fat.

youth givers

Carrots are possibly the most beneficial of anti-aging vegetables. As well as cleansing, nourishing and stimulating the whole body, their rich supply of betacarotene has been found to lower the risk of cancer – eating just one medium-sized carrot per day can halve the risk of lung cancer. Other orange vegetables such as pumpkin, squash and sweet potatoes are also high in betacarotene.

Avocados are a good source of monounsaturated fat, which may help the body to reduce levels of "bad" cholesterol. A good source of vitamin E, avocado can help prevent skin aging, and its rich potassium content staves off fluid retention and high blood pressure.

green vegetation

Broccoli, cauliflower, Brussels sprouts, cabbage and watercress supply a toxin- and cancer-fighting cocktail of phytochemicals, and stimulate the liver. Broccoli has a plentiful supply of many B and C vitamins, and minerals such as calcium, folate, iron, potassium and zinc, and spinach contains a vast amount of minerals and antioxidants.

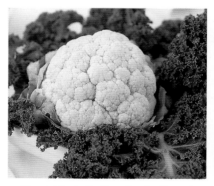

▲ Vegetables in the Brassica family, such as cauliflower, help to prevent cancer.

104 health-giving fish

Choosing from a variety of fish provides you with vital protein, minerals, vitamins and Omega 3 fatty acids. White fish is low in fat, while oily fishes such as tuna and mackerel are rich in vitamins A and D.

This tasty mackerel recipe is rich in Omega 3 fatty acids, which help prevent coronary heart disease and leave the skin clear and glowing.

moroccan spiced mackerel

serves 4

150ml/¹/₄ pint sunflower oil
15ml/1 tbsp paprika
5–10ml/1–2 tsp chilli powder
10ml/2 tsp ground cumin
10ml/2 tsp ground coriander
2 garlic cloves, crushed
juice of 2 lemons
salt and freshly ground black pepper
30ml/2 tbsp chopped mint leaves
30ml/2 tbsp chopped
　　coriander (cilantro) leaves
4 fresh mackerel, cleaned
mint sprigs, to garnish

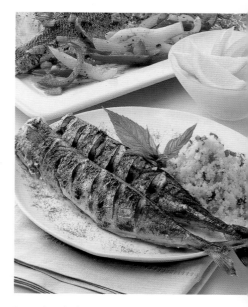

Whisk together the oil, spices, garlic and lemon juice. Season, then stir in the chopped mint and coriander to make a spicy marinade. Use a sharp knife to make a few diagonal slashes on either side of each mackerel.

Pour the marinade into a shallow non-metallic dish. Place the mackerel in the dish and spoon the marinade into the slashes, so that they absorb as much as possible. Cover the dish and leave to marinate for 3 hours. Preheat the grill to medium–high heat.

Transfer the fish to a rack set over a grilling pan and grill for 5–7 minutes, turning the fish once and basting several times. Serve the mackerel hot or cold, garnished with mint sprigs. Herb couscous or brown rice make good anti-aging accompaniments.

105 powerful proteins

Protein is essential for life, but only a very small amount is needed each day. Too much can contribute to a variety of health problems as you get older, including osteoporosis.

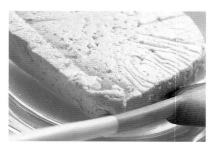

▲ *Soya products such as tofu can be cooked as nutritious meat substitutes.*

Most of us eat more protein that we need – estimates for requirements vary, but the range is from 5–10% of our total calorie intake. For best anti-aging results, try replacing at least some of your animal proteins with lower-fat plant proteins.

meat and poultry
Although red meat is a source of readily absorbed iron, zinc and B vitamins, it contains toxins, drugs and pesticides and is high in saturated fat. Eat only in moderation and choose lean cuts to reduce harmful fat intake. A good source of quality protein, B vitamins and iron, poultry is low in fat if the skin is removed, but should still be eaten sparingly. Choose organic, free-range poultry to ensure it is healthy, nutritious and cruelty-free.

dairy products
Yogurt is the most beneficial dairy product as it is non-mucus-forming and contains *Lactobacillus acidophilus*, which increases beneficial bacteria in the intestines and neutralizes excess hydrochloric acid in the stomach. Whole milk and cheese are mucus-forming (causing nasal congestion) and high in saturated fat, but may be consumed in moderation.

pulses
Beans and legumes such as lentils, pinto and mung beans, chick peas and soya beans are excellent sources of plant protein. Use dry beans in cooking, as processing, in all but a few exceptions, adds sugar and salt – they can be used to make delicious stews, soups and casseroles.

Tofu has been used in Chinese and Japanese cuisine for centuries – and the resulting reduction in saturated fats has been implicated in the lower incidence of cancers in these cultures.

106 fibre-rich grains

Providing fibre, carbohydrates, protein and minerals, grains have been a major part of the human diet for thousands of years. When eaten in whole form, they are potent anti-agers.

Eaten in moderation, grains are said to promote age reversal due to their rich supply of vitamins B and E, EFAs and lecithin, which helps to oxygenate the tissues. By absorbing impurities in the blood, fibre reduces levels of low-density lipoprotein and cholesterol levels, important in the prevention of heart disease.

Unprocessed whole grains, including brown rice, oats, barley, millet, rye, buckwheat and quinoa contain soluble and insoluble fibre, and are fundamental in preventing constipation, colon and rectal cancers. Research has shown that they also help prevent heart disease.

oat sense

An important anti-ager and easy to digest, a bowl of hot oats quickly helps cholesterol exit the body, and leaves the complexion glowing. Oats also act as a tonic for the nervous system, and stabilize sugar metabolism.

super sprouts

With their high nutrient level sprouted grains are the richest source of vitamins, minerals and enzymes – sprouted oats contain 1,000 times as much vitamin B as unsprouted.

▼ *Start the day with oat porridge and fruit for a supply of slow-burning energy.*

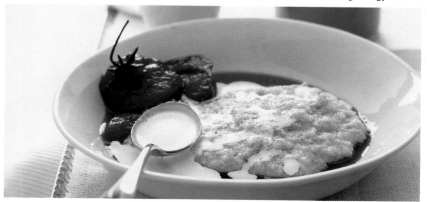

107 antioxidant juices

Juicing fresh fruits provides you with antioxidant enzymes that serve to protect your cells from damaging free radicals. For maximum benefit, drink the juice directly after preparing.

By drinking fresh juice, you will retain all the important youth-enhancing, antioxidant enzymes contained in the fruit. Excellent for kick-starting the digestive system, the following high-energy drink is delicious at breakfast. You may also wish to create your own blends from combinations of papaya, mango, cantaloupe melon and white, green or black grapes – all are very beneficial.

pink vitality
serves 1
1 peach or nectarine
225g/8oz strawberries
30ml/2tbsp lemon juice

Cut the peach or nectarine into quarters around the stone (pit) and pull the fruit apart. Cut the flesh into rough chunks, then hull the strawberries. Juice all the fruit using a juicer, or blend in a blender for a thick juice with pulp. Stir in the lemon juice and drink immediately.

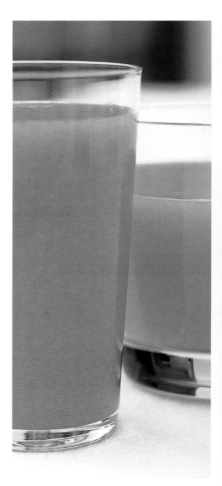

▸ *A blend of peach, strawberries and lemon juice makes a delicious drink rich in antioxidants.*

For a rejuvenating, caffeine-free beverage, steep a teaspoon of chamomile, peppermint, fennel or mixed spices in boiling water for five minutes. Strain and enjoy.

109 essential fats

Contrary to popular belief, it is important to eat a variety of fats daily. If you learn the difference between "good" and "bad" fats, your body will reap the benefits – now and in the future.

Choosing the right fat is important for sustaining vitality as the body ages. Plant oils provide essential fatty acids (EFAs) and vitamin E, beneficial for heart and skin. High in unsaturated fats, olive, sunflower and grapeseed oils are all good choices. Often called the "king of oils", olive oil's tried and tested benefits in the Mediterranean diet include protection against heart disease. Some essential substances are lost from oils that are heated during processing, so look for organic, extra virgin olive oil and cold-pressed oils.

fats to avoid
Saturated fats – butter, cream, meat fats, palm and coconut oils – should be eaten in moderation, as they can raise cholesterol levels and clog the arteries. Processed foods such as "fast foods", cakes and biscuits often use hydrogenated fats, which are also saturated and are linked with cancer.

Omega magic
Foods and supplements with essential fatty acids (EFAs) can make dramatic improvements to skin tone and joint flexibility. Supplements with fish or flax oils contain Omegas 3, 6 and 9, which help the skin produce new elastin and collagen, making it firmer and more youthful. High in gamma-linoleic acid (GLA), evening primrose oil helps to regulate the hormones and control rheumatoid arthritis.

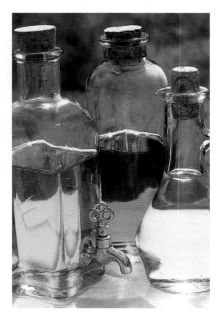

◄ *Cold-pressed oils, such as olive and sunflower, are best for the anti-aging dieter.*

110

mineral-packed nuts & seeds

Nuts and seeds have excellent, youth-preserving benefits, since they contain compact energy in the form of protein, fats, carbohydrates and myriad minerals. Include several types in your daily diet.

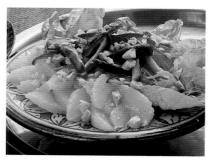

▲ For a mineral-rich addition to salads, throw in a handful of your favourite nuts.

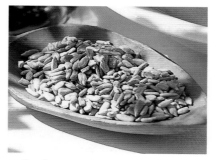

▲ Sunflower seeds are delicious and easy to carry for a quick afternoon pick-me-up.

go nuts

Most varieties of nuts are good sources of minerals, especially walnuts and brazil nuts. Although high in calories, walnuts are rich in iron, zinc, potassium, magnesium, copper and selenium. Almonds, peanuts, cashews, hazelnuts and pine nuts also offer excellent health benefits.

Adding nuts to your diet in small quantities can work to enhance the effectiveness of your digestive and immune systems and improve the quality of your skin and hair. Though high in fat, they actually help reduce cholesterol levels because the fat they contain is polyunsaturated.

Nuts stay fresh longer when bought in the shell and used as needed. They can be eaten on their own, or added to porridge, breads, casseroles and salads. Never eat rancid nuts – they have been linked to cancer-causing free radicals.

grab a seed snack

Seeds such as pumpkin, sunflower and sesame offer high nutritional values with slightly fewer calories than nuts. Sunflower seeds, for example, are a good source of vitamin B3 (niacin), known to fight depression, high blood pressure, circulatory problems and asthma. Add to breads and salads.

111 sulphur-rich eggs & garlic

An important protector against radiation and chemical pollutants, sulphur has also been shown to prolong the life span of animals. Eggs and garlic are both excellent sources.

amino acid protection

Sulphur-based amino acids such as methionine, cysteine and taurine are important antioxidant nutrients – they scavenge free radicals, neutralize toxic waste and help process proteins. They also help to protect against the effects of radiation from X-rays, mobile phones, power lines and low-level nuclear radiation, to which we are increasingly exposed.

food sources

As well as containing the most complete nutrition of any food – including protein, iron, zinc and

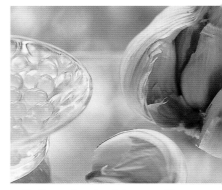

▲ Garlic may be taken in its natural form (cloves) or as a deodorized supplement.

▼ Fresh, free-range eggs are an excellent source of sulphur and many other nutrients.

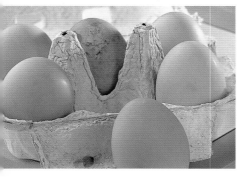

vitamins A, E and B complex – eggs are a rich source of sulphur, with 65mg each. The human body contains around 140g of sulphur and almost a gram is lost every day.

Garlic – like other members of the *Allium* family, such as onions – also contains a high level of sulphur. In addition, eating a clove of garlic a day (which may be raw or cooked) helps protect against heart disease – it reduces cholesterol levels and assists blood-thinning more effectively than aspirin, thus reducing the risk of heart attack and stroke.

112 cell-boosting vitamin C

Vitamin C is one of the most important nutrients in cell repair and therefore a potent anti-aging agent. Together with vitamin E and betacarotene, it is one of the "big three" antioxidants.

An essential nutrient for maintaining a resilient immune system, vitamin C assists with tissue growth, the healing of wounds, and the prevention of blood clotting and bruising. It is a powerful antioxidant which, when taken with betacarotene and vitamin E, helps curtail the effects of pollution. It reduces facial wrinkles and promotes a smooth complexion, due to its role in maintaining collagen, which binds cells together.

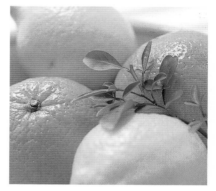

▲ Citrus fruits such as oranges are an important source of vitamin C.

▼ Versatile tomatoes contain a good supply of vitamin C and other antioxidants.

high–C foods and supplements

Vitamin C is ideally sourced from the food you eat, and many fruits and vegetables are high in it. Choose from a variety of berries, citrus fruits, kiwi fruits, green leafy vegetables, guavas, tomatoes, apples, melons and peppers to include in your daily diet.

When choosing supplements, try to find a brand with bioflavonoids, which work in conjunction with vitamin C. As it is not retained by the body, time–released vitamin C offers most benefit, allowing slow leaching into the digestive tract. Many health advisers recommend 200–500mg a day to keep infections at bay.

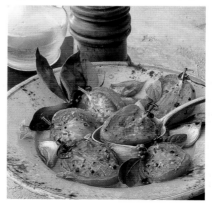

113 health-preserving vitamin E

Vitamin E is an essential fat-soluble substance containing several antioxidant compounds that help the body to fight free radicals and boost immunity to aid in the prevention of disease.

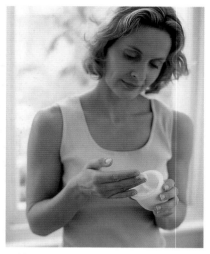

▲ *Vitamin E creams and oils help to heal burns and soothe dry, damaged skin.*

In laboratory tests, vitamin E has been shown to slow the aging process and enhance immune functions. Those with higher levels of this important antioxidant get fewer infections than people with average levels. Vitamin E is also known to help prevent degenerative diseases such as heart disease, arthritis, diabetes and cancer. It keeps your skin looking younger and glowing, and helps keep wrinkles at bay. Vitamin E deficiency is rare, but signs include thread veins and slow-healing wounds.

sources of vitamin E

Vitamin E is found in many foods: nuts, sunflower and pumpkin seeds, cold-pressed oils, vegetables, spinach, grains, asparagus, avocado, beef,

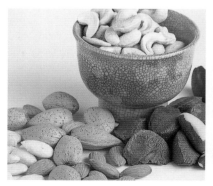

▲ *Nuts such as almonds and cashews are a good source of healing vitamin E.*

seafood, apples, carrots and celery. As a supplement, vitamin E is best taken with betacarotene, vitamin C and selenium. Experts recommend no more than 600–1,200IU daily. Always build up to higher doses slowly.

114 protective betacarotene

An important antioxidant in preventing age degeneration of the cells and tissues, betacarotene appears to fight several forms of cancer as well as offering many other benefits.

Betacarotene – or pro-vitamin A – is converted to vitamin A by the body from foods, but unlike vitamin A, it is not toxic in high doses. A plant substance, this antioxidant boosts the immune system and has been shown to slow many types of cancer.

In studies, it was shown that women who had eaten betacarotene-rich foods for 18 months had a lower

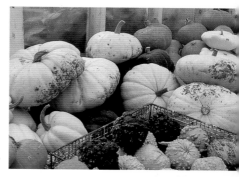

▲ Pumpkins and the many varieties of squash are rich sources of betacarotene.

risk of cancer – but those who benefited most had been eating these foods for 20 years or more.

beta benefits

Betacarotene promotes growth and strong bones; it strengthens teeth, hair, skin and gums and helps the respiratory systems resist infections. It also helps prevent night blindness and improves weak eyesight.

It is found in many fruits and vegetables, including carrots, pumpkins, squashes, spinach, broccoli, cantaloupe, sweet potatoes, apricots, peaches, Brussels sprouts and oranges.

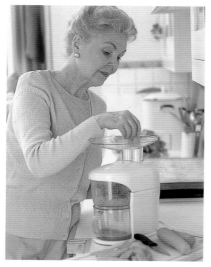

▼ Carrots have been found to reduce the risk of breast cancer after the menopause.

115

essential B & K vitamins

Because of their role in releasing energy from food, providing the body with steady nutrients, B group and K vitamins are vital. Eat a range of vitamin B-rich foods, as they work in tandem with each other.

the B group

When adopting a balanced anti-aging diet, consuming a variety of foods that contain all of the B vitamins is important. B group vitamins are found in large quantities in liver and yeast, and they exist singly or in combinations in all of the food groups. Eat seeds, nuts, legumes, dairy products, meats, fish and eggs.

Vitamins B6, B12 and folate are important in staving off the effects of aging, because they affect methylation, an essential chemical process that helps maintain the body's DNA and protein. They are also believed to

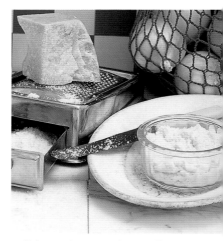

▲ *Dairy products contain many B group vitamins; yogurt is also rich in vitamin K.*

▼ *Nuts, legumes and seeds such as pumpkin all contain B complex vitamins.*

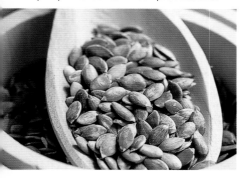

protect the heart and brain from age-related damage, balance the hormones and prevent depression.

the K concept

Vitamin K has excellent anti-aging properties. It is believed to reduce the risk of osteoporosis, improve bone health, strengthen gums and reduce the risk of heart disease. Sources include broccoli, Brussels sprouts, liver, yogurt, beans, soya and lean red meat.

116 bone-protecting calcium

Important for strong bones and teeth, adequate amounts of calcium and vitamin D help prevent the onset of osteoporosis, one of the most significant age-related illnesses, especially in women.

calcium count

Eating a diet that is rich in calcium is invaluable in protecting the body from osteoporosis – a disease in which the bones become fragile and brittle. It is important to start as young as possible – fortifying the body with plenty of calcium in the teenage years and young adulthood can reduce the risk of developing the disease in later years.

Foods that contain rich supplies of calcium include almonds, sesame seeds, beans, tofu and dairy products such as milk, cheese and yogurt. Other foods that offer good supplies include fish such as sprats, whitebait and sardines, particularly when their bones are eaten as well as the flesh.

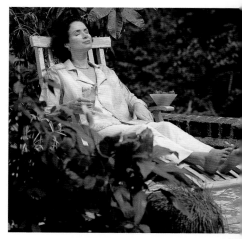

▲ *Spending time in the sunlight will ensure that your body receives enough vitamin D.*

THE SUNLIGHT VITAMIN

Vitamin D is also crucial for strong bones, and some exposure to sunlight is essential for boosting body supplies. Extra vitamin D can be obtained from sea fish such as salmon, sardines and herring, from fish liver oils and egg yolks, or by taking it in tablet form.

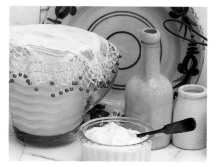

◀ *Dairy products such as milk, yogurt and cheese are good sources of calcium.*

117 super antioxidants

Grapeseed extract and tea polyphenols are antioxidants with strong life-preserving qualities. You can get your supply by eating grapes and drinking tea, or by taking supplements.

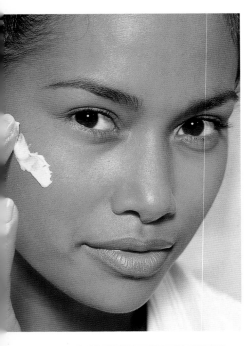

grapeseed extract

A bioflavonoid that acts to keep capillaries and connective tissue in good condition, grapeseed extract is a potent free radical scavenger. It is very beneficial for smokers, those exposed to second-hand smoke and exercisers, all of whom are bombarded by free radicals (exercisers are at risk due to their faster metabolisms). You can chew on the seeds of white or green grapes, or take supplements.

tea polyphenols

Due to its high polyphenol content, green tea is a goldmine of cancer-fighting properties. Polyphenols seem to deter cancer in three ways: they stop the cancer cells from forming, increase the body's detoxification defenses, and prevent cancer cells from growing. They also act as skin detoxifiers and skin-aging inhibitors.

Black tea contains about half the polyphenol content of green tea, but is still useful drunk in small quantities. White tea, which is dried in sunlight and is very expensive, has the highest level of polyphenols of all the teas – about three times that of green tea.

COSMETIC MAGIC
In addition to ingesting these antioxidants, using them externally also helps protect the skin from damage. Many commercial skin ranges use tea polyphenols and grapeseed extract in their moisturizers and cosmetics.

118

herbal brain boosters

Ginkgo biloba and vinpocetine are natural plant substances that are used therapeutically to boost brain power and delay the onset of age-related memory loss and other problems.

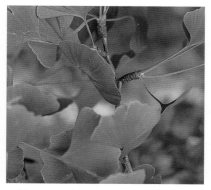

▲ *Memory-enhancing ginkgo biloba.*

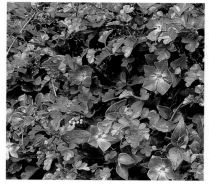

▲ *The periwinkle provides vinpocetine.*

ginkgo biloba

The earliest known medicinal use of ginkgo – often called "The Fountain of Youth" because the plant has survived 200 million years – dates back to 2800BC. Today it is one of the most popular herbal remedies in the world, due largely to its role in improving brain function. Ginkgo is used to combat memory loss, and to treat the early stages of Alzheimer's disease and depression in the elderly. This amazing plant also aids poor circulation, erectile problems and hearing loss, and it is used as a long-term therapy for stroke victims.

vinpocetine

Derived from the periwinkle plant, the action of vinpocetine is similar to that of gingko biloba. It works to improve mental function by increasing the blood circulation to the brain, thus improving the way the brain uses glucose and oxygen. It also enhances the function of neurotransmitters such as serotonin, which regulates emotions, mood, sleep and appetite. (Serotonin levels often fall when people are under stress.) Vinpocetine guards against ear problems such as tinnitus (ringing in the ears) and vertigo (dizziness).

119 age-defying supplements

Certain substances occur naturally in the body, but either exist in small quantities or their production declines from an early age. Supplements can provide dramatic anti-aging effects.

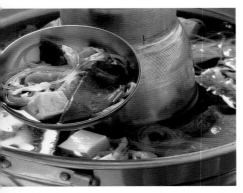

▲ *Supplements are a good way to boost levels of co-enzyme Q-10 and carnosine.*

co-enzyme Q-10

This super-nutrient, also called ubiquinone, is an antioxidant with a huge number of anti-aging benefits. Its most important effects include lowering blood pressure, boosting the immune system, protecting the brain and eyes from damage, and helping to prevent heart disease.

Co-enzyme Q-10 fights aging at the mitochondrial level in the cells, and may dramatically reverse the effects of aging and a poor diet. Although it is a natural substance made by the body, the production of co-enzyme Q-10 declines around the age of 20, and many people take it as a supplement. Food sources include trout, sardines, mackerel, nuts and soya.

carnosine

An antioxidant amino acid found in brain, muscle and eye tissue, carnosine stabilizes and protects cell membranes, and scavenges free radicals from both external pollutants and internal chemical reactions. It helps fight the process of glycosylation – a dangerous coupling of sugar molecules to body protein – which causes widespread damage and aging. Food sources include lean red meat and chicken.

▼ *Co-enzyme Q-10 is present in small amounts in mackerel and other oily fish.*

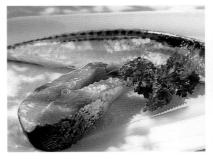

By eating just three or four **brazil nuts** a day, you will get your quota of **selenium**, which helps to prevent cancer and may **extend** life.

121 yoga for flexibility

Anti-aging experts agree that yoga is the top exercise for promoting longevity. It fosters balance, control and peace of mind, and lends the body great suppleness and fluidity.

Yoga works to build up a store of physical health, while keeping the body and mind cleansed and fit. The asanas (exercises) help in the removal of toxins, circulation of the blood and the smooth function of the organs.

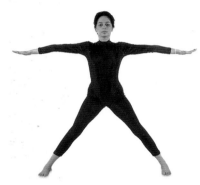

1 To perform the Warrior, stand with your feet together and arms at your side. Inhale deeply and jump the feet 120cm/4ft apart. Extend the arms.

2 Turn the palms up and stretch your arms over your head. Keep the arms parallel, elbows tight and palms facing each other.

3 Turn right leg 45° in, and left foot 90° out, turning hips to the left. Bring right hip forwards and left hip slightly back.

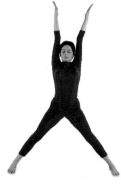

4 Exhale; bend left leg into a right angle, stretching whole body. Take head back and stretch for 20–30 seconds. Repeat.

122 heart-enhancing aerobics

The benefits of aerobic exercise are many, but the most important for anti-aging is its very positive effect on the heart and cardiovascular system, keeping the body fit and "tuned".

Any exercise that increases the respiratory rate and boosts the heart rate from 60–80% of its capacity is called aerobic, meaning "sustained by oxygen". Tennis, jogging, cycling, dancing and swimming are all excellent aerobic sports. Perhaps the easiest and most accessible is walking: it can be done anywhere, needs no special equipment and varies endlessly with different locations and terrains. Aerobics classes with planned routines are available at most night schools and gyms, and some target specific age groups and fitness levels.

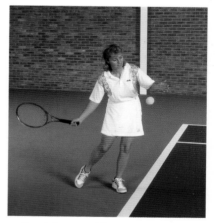

▲ Tennis is an aerobic activity that can be enjoyed in the fresh air with a friend.

powerful advantages

Aerobic exercise burns fat, boosts the immune system and helps prevent the build-up of fatty deposits in the arteries. It enhances joint and muscle flexibility, and aids stamina, digestion and sleep – if you suffer at all from insomnia, this is your first port of call for a remedy. The body was designed for movement, and if it doesn't move, all of its systems suffer. The mind suffers too; exercise is a major ingredient in keeping mentally fit as well as physically active.

never too late

Recent studies have shown that even people who have not exercised for 20 years can benefit significantly from an aerobics regime. It is possible to gain the fitness levels of a younger body in a surprisingly short period of time, and the sooner you start, the sooner you will reap the rewards. Begin slowly, gradually building up your stamina, strength and suppleness. Consult your doctor if you are planning to start exercising after years of inactivity.

123 retaining youth through yoga

Many yoga positions can help you stay fresh and youthful. Try a Forward Bend when you need to calm down and relax, while a Lighting Bolt will give you a dynamic surge of energy.

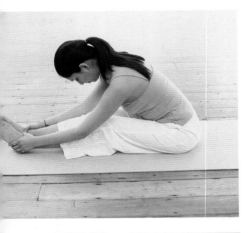

seated forward bend

Sit upright on your tailbone, with your legs together and straight out in front of you, toes up. On an outbreath, fold forwards from the hips to hold your ankles or your toes, without hunching your back. Ideally, keep your legs straight and bring your head down towards your knees, but let your knees bend if your back hurts, and don't force yourself to reach further than is comfortable. Hold for up to 30 seconds, then slowly return, on an in breath, to an upright sitting position.

lightning bolt

1 Stand with your feet hip-width apart and your arms to the sides. Breathe in as you raise your arms above your head. Breathe out and bend your knees so that they are directly above your toes. Be careful not to let your knees buckle inwards.

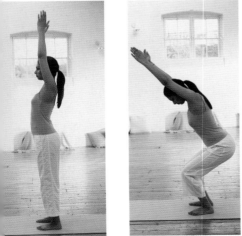

2 Extend the arms in line wih your torso. Breathe deeply three or four times, feeling the energy of the lightning bolt that your body forms from fingertips to toes. On an in breath, return to your starting position.

safe lifting

As you get older, innocent, everyday tasks can be a minefield of potential injuries. With a little care, movements such as bending, squatting, sitting, standing and lifting can be performed safely.

Back problems become increasingly common with age and inactivity, and many injuries are brought on by incorrect movement. This exercise will help you to retrain your body to support the lower back while bending and lifting loads. To avoid unnecessary strain on the back, stand as close to the load as possible and place your feet to either side of it.

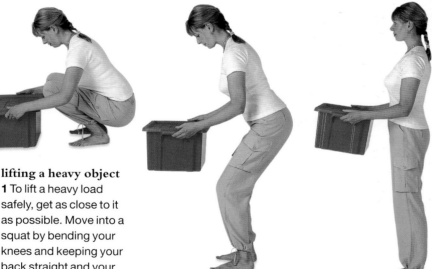

lifting a heavy object
1 To lift a heavy load safely, get as close to it as possible. Move into a squat by bending your knees and keeping your back straight and your feet firmly on the ground. Keep your head aligned with your back bone. Bend your arms so that your elbows are close to your body to help you lift.

2 Hold the load firmly without tensing the wrists. If the arms, wrists and hands are tense, you will lose the contact with your lower back.

3 Once you are holding the load as closely to your body as possible, slowly rise out of the squat and stand.

125 natural face lift

Tension held in the face can lead to wrinkles and sagging muscles as gravity comes into effect. By doing simple exercises each day, you can help retain the youthful elasticity of your features.

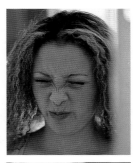

line eraser
1 Scrunch up your whole face for a few seconds, so that your nose is wrinkled, your forehead furrowed, and your eyes and mouth are tightly closed.

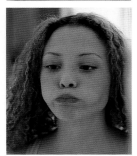

2 Now do the opposite: open your mouth and eyes as wide as you can (as if you are silently screaming) to release the tension in your throat and neck muscles.

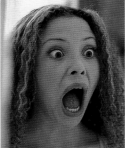

3 Relax your eyes for a moment. Close your mouth again, purse your lips and push your mouth up first to the left, and then to the right.

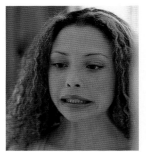

4 Grin widely and open your eyes wide. Relax the eyes, hold and repeat the grin, this time tucking your chin in. Relax and repeat once more.

CHIN FIRMER
Using the backs of your hands alternately, pat the area beneath your chin using quick, stroking movements. Done for a few minutes every day, this will help to firm up slack skin and reduce signs of a double chin.

126 abdomen strengthener

The girdle of muscles in the abdomen supports the spine and torso. To keep fit, healthy and free from back pain, it is important to keep this area toned and strong with simple exercises.

When doing these sit-ups, lift your head and shoulders as one unit, never separately – roll up from the top of your head. It may help to imagine that you are holding a peach between your chin and chest, and try to keep this gap constant throughout. Be sure to keep your facial muscles relaxed and loose.

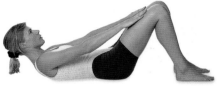

sit-ups

1 Lying flat on the floor with your arms by your sides and your palms down, bend your knees and keep your feet flat on the floor, a short distance apart and in line with your hips. Be sure to keep your lower abdomen tight by keeping the muscles contracted throughout the exercise.

2 Lift your head and shoulders upwards, exhaling as you rise, and push your fingertips towards your knees, keeping your arms straight.

NOTE
With any exercise, is important to stop if you feel anything more than a mild sensation of muscle fatigue. Always work at your own pace and stop if you feel dizzy. Do not attempt to exercise when you are ill or feverish.

3 Lower your body back to the starting position, breathing in as you go down. When you get to the floor, do not allow yourself a chance to rest but repeat the movement from step 1.

balancing t'ai chi

An ancient martial art and active meditation, t'ai chi is practised daily by millions of Chinese – many very long-lived. It enhances balance and has a "grounding" effect on the nervous system.

The physical and mental aspects of t'ai chi are very closely entwined. In Chinese medicine and philosophy, the interdependence of mind, body and spirit is seen as crucial for one's well-being. In t'ai chi, the alertness, relaxed mind, softening and opening of the joints, balance and flow of chi (energy) evenly through the body are all equally important.

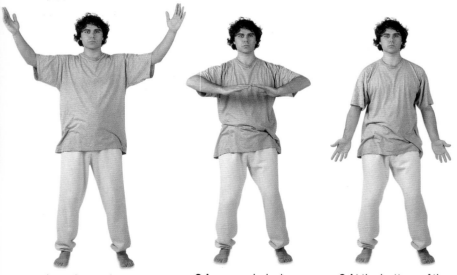

return to centre
1 As you breathe in, move your hands out to the sides in front of your body, and raise them slowly in a large circle, palms facing upwards.

2 As you exhale, lower your hands in front of the centre of your body, with your palms facing downwards.

3 At the bottom of the circle, turn your hands outwards again to begin a new circle with the new breath. Repeat several times until the movement is flowing.

128 deep breathing exercises

Proper breathing is important for a youthful system. It facilitates the movement of oxygen through the blood, "feeding" the cells, removing impurities and enhancing the body's energy flow.

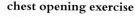

chest opening exercise

1 These exercises help to open up the chest to better facilitate deep breathing. Stand with your feet shoulder-width apart and your knees bent. Lift your arms out to the sides with your elbows bent, and make loose fists with your hands. Take a deep breath in, opening your chest by bringing your arms back as much as possible.

2 On exhaling, cross your arms in front of you, and relax your head down. Keeping your knees bent, press the area in between your shoulder blades backwards, and feel the muscles stretching. Empty your breath out completely. Repeat the exercise 4 or 5 times.

lung stretch

Link your index fingers and thumbs. Step forward with your right foot and reach up to the ceiling. Look up as you breathe in, and feel your chest expanding as your lungs fill with air.

Step back with your foot and relax your arms as you breathe out. Step forward again, this time with your left foot, and repeat the same movement. Repeat another 3 or 4 times.

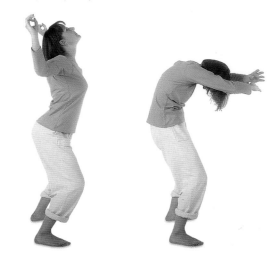

129 nourishing night cream

As the body matures, the skin becomes drier and loses elasticity. Moisturizing at night with a rich cream can help your face retain its youthful smoothness and rounded contours.

The delicate skin of the face is constantly exposed to the elements. To keep fine lines at bay, try this cosmetic, which uses a perfume-free base cream rich in vitamin E or evening primrose oil.

Jasmine and rose oils are added to help rehydrate the skin, while the frankincense oil helps to reduce wrinkles and restore tone to slack muscles. Good-quality essential oils can be obtained from health food stores, and there are many brands of prepared creams available.

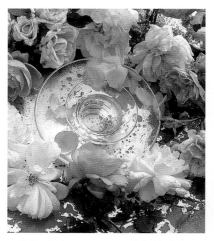

▲ Not only does rose essential oil help to rejuvenate the skin, its scent is heavenly.

▼ Use night cream only on cleansed skin or you will trap impurities, which can irritate.

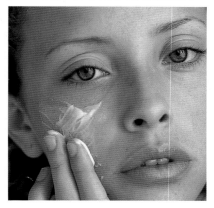

nourishing night cream

50g/2oz jar of unperfumed vitamin E
  or evening primrose oil cream
3 drops rose essential oil
2 drops frankincense essential oil
1 drop jasmine essential oil

Add the oils to the cream and mix with a clean metal spoon. After washing, apply small dabs to the forehead, cheeks, chin, nose and neck. Massage gently into the skin.

For a sensual treat, use 1 tablespoon almond oil plus 3 drops each rose and sandalwood oils, swirl into a warm bath and climb into a youthful indulgence.

131 gentle eye treatments

Tired, puffy eyes can occur for many reasons – computer fatigue, lack of sleep or crying – making you appear older. These home-made remedies will refresh the delicate eye area and reduce swelling.

The following treatments involve lying down with your eyes closed for at least 15 minutes. This relaxation period is almost as important a part of the treatment as the compresses.

▾ *Tea contains astringent tannin, making it ideal for a simple compress for tired eyes.*

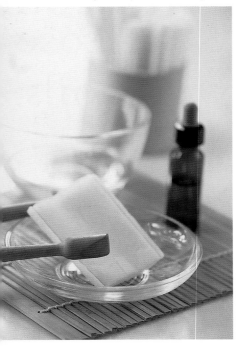

cooling cucumber

Place a cool slice of fresh organic cucumber over each eye and then relax. Cucumber works very gently to tone and refresh the skin around the eyes while reducing swelling.

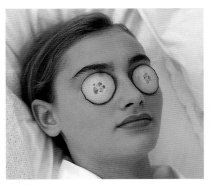

tea bag treatment

Ordinary tea contains tannin, which is astringent and tones the skin. Place a couple of Indian or African tea bags on a saucer and pour hot water over them. Cover with another saucer and refrigerate until cool. Gently squeeze the excess moisture from the bags, place them over your eyes, lie down and relax. Remove the tea bags and gently pat the skin dry before dabbing on a gentle moisturizer.

132 restorative hair mask

As hair ages, it tends to become drier and more brittle, especially grey hair that has been colour-treated. Applying a hair mask will help restore moisture and gloss to tired hair.

Deep conditioning of the hair will help promote shiny, lustrous locks. For a really rich, moisturizing treatment that adds body to dry or lank hair, try the following once every two or three weeks. As the ingredients are all natural, the preparation is safe to use even on tinted hair.

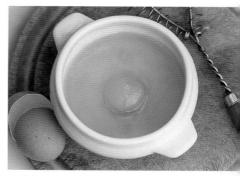

rich hair mask
1 egg yolk, lightly beaten
15ml/1tbsp olive oil

Beat ingredients together. Work the mask into dry hair before washing and massage into the scalp. Gently comb or finger through, then wrap in a warm towel; leave for 20–30 minutes. Follow with a gentle shampoo, using a a final rinse of cool water.

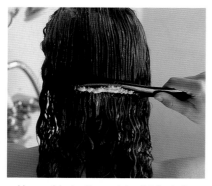

▲ *Use a wide-tooth comb to distribute the conditioner evenly through the strands.*

GREYING
At some stage during middle adulthood, the pigment formation in hair slows down and silver-grey strands begin to appear. The speed of the process is largely due to genetic factors, but foods containing vitamin B5 are said to help slow the onset of grey hair. Eating a wide selection of fruit, vegetables and nuts will ensure your hair is kept in optimum condition, whatever its colour.

133 skin sense

The youngest-looking people are those who eat fresh foods, drink plenty of water and shun the midday sun. Not only is this wise from a vanity point of view, it also helps prevent skin cancer.

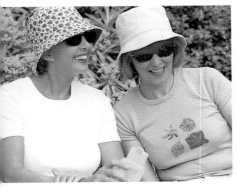

▲ Sun hats help prevent damage to skin.

As skin ages, it loses collagen and becomes drier, more "brittle" and thin, factors that lead to fine lines and wrinkles. The skin on the hands and face age faster due to exposure to the elements and pollutants, but there are ways that you can slow the process.

avoid UV light and smoke
The single most effective way to prevent premature skin aging is to protect your skin from the UV (ultraviolet) rays of the sun. Although a little sunshine is no bad thing, particularly as the body needs it to manufacture vitamin D, when out in bright sunlight, it is best to wear a hat and sunglasses, and use a sunscreen with an SPF (Sun Protection Factor) of at least 15, depending on your skin colour and type.

healthy tips
Water is important for healthy skin – it flushes out toxins and moisturizes from the inside. When skin is exposed to artificial heat in buildings, it can lose up to 2 litres/3 $^1/2$ pints of water per day, so keep rehydrating. Eat fresh foods rich in vitamins A, C and E, betacarotene, selenium and zinc, and get good quality sleep each night.

FACIAL MOISTURIZING
There are a number of good facial creams and lotions available commercially, and constant advances in research mean that these often contain many of the latest known anti-aging ingredients, vitamins and antioxidants. Products containing alpha-hydroxy acids (AHAs) are said to combat some of the effects of aging by "sloughing off" the top layers of epidermis.

134 soothing hand cream

The hands are the most used part of the body – they tend to age faster due to exposure to water, detergent and the elements. This lotion will help heal and protect against chapped, dry skin.

Lavender contains over 200 active substances, and is perfect for use in moisturizers as it not only soothes and heals, but has a wonderful fragrance as well. By making your own hand cream, you ensure that the ingredients are fresh and free from chemical additives and preservatives. The materials needed for this recipe are available from most chemists.

▾ *Lavender hand cream acts as a rejuvenating barrier that fights dryness caused by exposure to pollutants.*

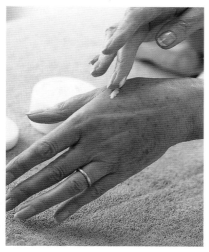

lavender moisturizer
20g/³/₄oz cocoa butter
10ml/2tsp borax
175ml/6fl oz lavender water
75ml/5tbsp almond oil
20ml/4tsp beeswax granules
8 drops lavender essential oil
mixing bowl
saucepans
wooden spoon
glass jar

Measure out the cocoa butter, borax, lavender water, almond oil and beeswax granules in separate containers. Put the beeswax, cocoa butter and almond oil in a bowl set over a saucepan of simmering water. Stir well until the ingredients melt.

In a separate pan, dissolve the borax and lavender water by gently warming it. Add the lavender/borax mixture to the bowl; stir constantly. When the ingredients are thoroughly combined, take the mixture off the heat and allow it to cool. While still tepid, add the lavender oil and mix well. Pour the moisturizer into a glass jar and store in the refrigerator. Use within three weeks.

135 invigorating aromatherapy

Aromatherapy oils work by sending molecules to the brain's olfactory centre via the nostrils, or by being absorbed into the skin. They can have significant physiological and psychological effects.

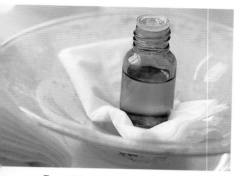

▲ Essential oils have many uses, from antidepressant to digestive stimulant.

anti-aging oils

Although there are no magic potions that will keep you young forever, certain plant essences can stimulate the growth of healthy new cells. The most effective are neroli and lavender.

Lavender is not only a powerful skin rejuvenator, it also helps balance both dry and greasy skins, and combats acne. Delicate neroli oil is used in many skincare products and is useful for dry and sensitive skin. It can also help the skin's elasticity, and improve the appearance of thread veins (common on older, thinner skin) and stretch marks.

oil dispersion

Essential oils can be used in a number of ways. Try placing a few drops in an oil burner to disperse throughout the room, or place on a tissue and sniff. You could also place a lightly impregnated piece of cloth or tissue inside your pillowcase at night.

Regular use of both lavender and neroli in baths and massage can help to maintain cellular reproduction at levels that naturally occur in younger people. Add a few drops of the oils to a very warm bath, or to a base oil such as almond for a relaxing massage. You can also experiment by adding the oils to face creams and body lotions.

OTHER USEFUL OILS
- **Rose** Antidepressant, sexual tonic, aphrodisiac.
- **Ylang ylang** Circulatory and respiratory stimulant, antispasmodic.
- **Black pepper** Analgesic, antidepressant, expectorant.
- **Ginger** Anticatarrhal, analgesic, digestive stimulant.
- **Myrrh** Anti-inflammatory, antiseptic, emotional sedative.

136 regenerative hydrotherapy

Water has been used as a healing aid throughout the centuries, in all cultures. By using hot or cold ablutions – or a combination – you can stimulate, cleanse and regenerate the body's systems.

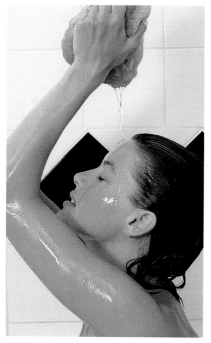

◀ *Cool, running water tightens and tones the skin and refreshes the whole body.*

vitality shower

Start by priming your body with a brief warm shower, until you feel the heat permeating your skin, but not so hot that you turn lobster red (very hot water damages skin tissue). Now turn on the cold tap, and direct the shower all over your body, from your face to your limbs, and down your torso and back, for 20–30 seconds.

Get out and pat yourself dry, then put on some warm clothes. If you cannot warm up afterwards, take another warm shower – do not risk giving yourself a chill.

anti-aging face affusion

Running water on the face stimulates the blood supply to the skin, leaving it more taut and fresh. Start by making sure your whole body is warm. Take the head off a shower attachment, and run cold water. Bending over the bath, rest your head on a rolled-up towel and let the stream of water flow gently over your face, in a circular motion, for three minutes. Pat dry.

As anyone who bathes in an open-air swimming pool knows, cold water is a wonderful tonic for the skin, leaving it glowing and healthy-looking. The positive stress of temperature change can make your immune system stronger and more resistant to illness, while giving you an energizing boost.

137 "spring clean" fast

Fasting is recommended by many anti-aging experts to cleanse the body, stimulate its systems and give the digestion a rest. This weekend fast is a gentle yet effective way to rejuvenate.

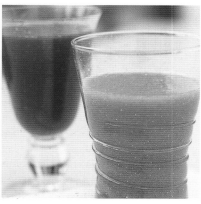

▲ Fresh juice contains healing enzymes.

People who fast periodically have been shown to have the tissues of a much younger body. Even after a short fast, improvements can be seen: facial lines soften, skin condition improves and eyes become brighter.

In this regime, plentiful fluids are combined with vegetables and fruits to rid the system of built-up impurities. Choose a weekend when you can allow yourself plenty of time for rest, relaxation and reflection. Book a massage and take some gentle exercise to stimulate the metabolism.

the fast

The evening before the fast, have a light, vegetable-based meal, such as soup or a green salad.

mornings

On rising, drink a cup of hot water with lemon juice to kick-start the liver. Prepare a fruit juice and dilute with water for breakfast. Eat a bunch of grapes or an apple mid-morning.

afternoons

Make up a fresh vegetable juice, such as carrot and spinach, and a large salad for lunch and drink plenty of mineral water. Do simple stretches all day.

evenings

Prepare a dinner of lightly steamed organic vegetables, sprinkled with fresh herbs and lemon juice, accompanied by brown rice. It is a good idea to end each day with relaxation techniques or meditation, followed by a warming bath.

Always consult a doctor or nutritionist if you plan a fast lasting longer than two days.

138 coping with depression

The likelihood of depression may increase as you get older, but there are ways to combat "feeling down". Recognizing the warning signs can help you take self-help action sooner.

Depression is different from the unhappy mood you may have when something goes wrong in your life. It is longer lasting and can affect your behaviour, relationships, sleeping and eating patterns, and your whole attitude towards living.

Events that can trigger depression include the breakup of a relationship, the death of a loved one and losing a job. Sometimes it has no specific cause, but may occur in older people due to a perceived loss of control in life. The prospect of aging may in itself be a cause of depression, especially in societies that are youth-orientated.

▼ Consider seeking help from a therapist if depression lingers for more than two weeks.

self-help

If you are feeling depressed, ensure that you continue to eat and sleep properly, and that your diet is high in C and B vitamins, essential fatty acids and unrefined carbohydrates. Avoid relying on bad habits such as drinking and drugs – they are false friends.

Exercise regularly – endorphins released during physical activity can help combat depression. Herbalists recommend taking St. John's wort tablets; aromatherapists value rose, neroli, clary sage and bergamot oils.

Don't be afraid to talk to friends and family. Try to explore with them your anxieties, anger and sadness. It is always easier to cope with problems when you can talk about them.

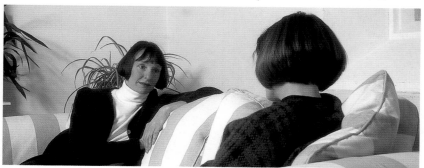

139 re-addressing stress

Stress can chip away stealthily at your health and happiness. Learning how to deal with it successfully will help you towards a lengthy and more satisfying life.

Research has shown that stress can have a profound impact on your health. Stress triggers the "fight or flight" syndrome, in which the body acts as though it is in a life-or-death situation. In this state of physiological arousal, the heartbeat and blood pressure are elevated, and stress hormones such as adrenaline rage through the bloodstream.

If you are constantly under stress, these factors will in time wear down your immune system, making you more susceptible to illness and disease – from common colds to cardio-vascular problems and even cancer.

relaxation techniques

Learning relaxation techniques is a powerful antidote to stress. Yoga and meditation help you to centre your thoughts and quiet the mind. Deep breathing helps to oxygenate the cells and relax muscles. Good therapies for releasing tension include massage and aromatherapy. A quick way to beat stress is to go for a walk – exercise uses up adrenaline and brings an endorphin rush that raises the mood, giving a sense of perspective.

re-train your thinking

Trying to think rationally about the causes of stress and anxiety can be helpful. It is often your perception of a situation that makes it stressful, and changing the way you view it can be extremely beneficial.

Make a list of practical things you can do to alleviate a problem, and a list of things that you cannot change. If you have done all that you can, give yourself a break from worry – remind yourself there is no point in fretting.

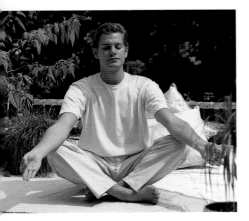

◀ *Take a deep breath and meditate on the causes of stress and how you can remedy it.*

140 satisfying sex

Important throughout adulthood, sexual activity can be a source of great pleasure, emotional nourishment and spiritual growth. Physical touch brings a confidence that extends to other areas.

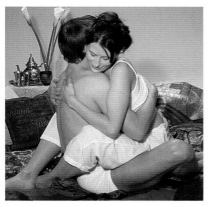

▲ *The intimacy that loving sex brings can provide a solid foundation for happiness.*

increased pleasure

Many people enjoy sex more as they get older, because they have gained experience and confidence. They understand what arouses them and their partner, and are more relaxed about communicating their desires.

The physical changes in sexuality vary. Most people do not notice any major changes until their 50s, when they may experience slower response times. One thing sex researchers agree on is the "use it or lose it" theory – staying sexually active keeps your sex organs functioning and helps maintain sexual desire.

getting closer

To keep long-term relationships alive and meaningful, try exploring different ways to arouse your partner, perhaps using visual stimuli, massage and aromatherapy. Learning about sexual philosophy and technique from different cultures can open deeply fulfilling doors. Tantric sex, from Eastern tradition, takes a holistic view of love and sex where the ultimate aim is for two people to merge spiritually as well as physically.

Touch is one of the most profound means of communication between two people. The laying of caring hands on the body conveys a depth of feeling that goes way beyond words – it is a direct link to the inner world of feeling, and through it you can express your innermost emotions and desires. People who live with one special partner for a long period – whether married or not – tend to be healthier and live longer. This is partly due to the benefits that regular, loving sex and physical intimacy bring.

141 nourishing sleep

Sleep is essential for physical and mental well-being. Although its pattern and quality may change as the body ages, it is an ever-important ingredient for youthfulness and health.

Deep sleep has a tremendous effect on vitality levels. It rejuvenates every cell in the body while resting the nervous system, which in turn is responsible for controlling the digestive, reproductive and immune systems. During sleep, not only are toxins eliminated and tissues rebuilt, but it is believed that the mind works through and helps resolve feelings, problems and challenges through the process of dreaming.

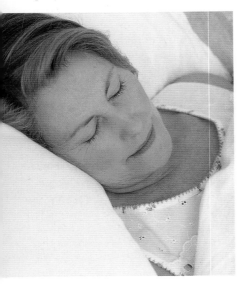

sleep patterns

Our sleep cycle is broken up into several distinct phases. Each of these is characterized by physiological activities such as eye movements and muscle tension, and the frequency of brain rhythms, or waves.

When we drop off to sleep we fall into "slow-wave" sleep, when the electrical activity of the brain slows down, together with our breathing and heart rate. Slow-wave sleep goes through four stages, with stage 1 at the earliest phase of sleep and stage 4 at the deepest, when the brainwaves are slowest. This is the time when it is most difficult to rouse someone.

After about 90 minutes of slow-wave sleep, Rapid Eye Movement (REM) sleep begins. The brainwaves speed up, heart and breathing rates increase, blood pressure rises and the eyes dart around behind closed lids. REM sleep is also called "dreaming sleep", as this is when we have our most vivid dreams – or at least those that we remember.

◀ *Sleep patterns change with age – try to discover what schedule works best for you.*

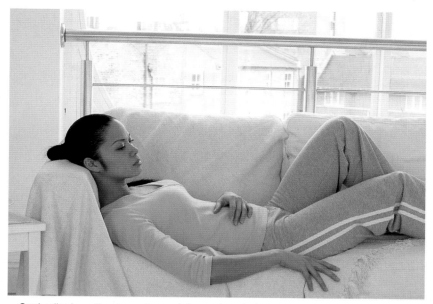

▲ *Our bodies have the chance to repair themselves during a good night's sleep. Insomnia affects us deeply and can make us irritable and moody.*

when do we dream?

It was once thought that dreams only occurred during repetitive eye movement (REM) sleep, but the development of science and the use of sleep laboratories has enabled researchers to study dreamers and their brain activity more closely. Gradually it transpired that dreams occur throughout the night during periods of non-REM sleep, although they are less vivid and usually forgotten.

aiding quality sleep

To ensure a deep and restful sleep, the two most important factors are good nutrition and proper exercise. It is best to refrain from caffeine, alcohol and excessive sugar in the evenings – these all exacerbate restlessness and

insomnia. Make sure that your bedroom environment is pleasant; that you have a firm bed, fresh air, clean bedclothes and quiet. It can help to take a hot bath an hour before bed; deep breathing and certain yoga poses will also help calm the nervous system.

changing sleep patterns

People may find it more difficult to sleep as they get older, possibly due to the body producing fewer chemicals that control the sleep cycle. Some find that they wake more frequently during the night and spend more time being awake. You can adapt to these natural changes by trying "sleepy" herbal teas before going to bed, or by taking a short nap in the afternoon to augment the sleep cycle.

142 healing natural light

Without the sun, there would be no life on Earth – people, plants and animals all move to the rhythm of its rays. Time spent outdoors will keep you in tune with the sun's healing energy.

Light impulses do not go just to the visual cortex in the brain. Some nerves go from the retina directly to the hypothalamus, a small organ that regulates most of the life-sustaining functions of the body, such as control of the autonomic nervous system, energy levels, internal temperature, cycles of rest and activity, growth, circulation, breathing, reproduction and the emotions. The hypothalamus directly affects the pituitary gland, which is the major controlling organ for the endocrine system and all its hormonal secretions. Light from the eyes also directly affects the pineal gland, which modifies our behaviour patterns according to the amount of light it receives. This pea-sized gland regulates our energy so that we can remain in balance with our environment.

Without sufficient exposure to the full colour spectrum in sunlight, the finely balanced chemical reactions in the body tend to falter, leaving it prone to ill health. Spending time outside every day will renew your stamina and raise your spirits.

▲ Time spent in the sun energizes the body.

LIVE OUTSIDE
It has been recommended that people spend at least twenty minutes outside in direct sunlight every day. If you wear glasses or contact lenses it is also a good idea to remove them for five or ten minutes every few hours, in order to get the benefit of natural light. Remember to always apply sun cream.

dawn to dusk

Experiments have shown that, as the sun rises, its red light increases the pulse, blood pressure and breathing rates: stimulating the body into alertness. These functions are further increased in orange light and reach their peak in yellow light when the sun is high in the sky. Similarly, when the sky turns to subduing blues and greens at dusk, the vital signs decrease and the body prepares for relaxation and sleep.

modern hazard

Many people have jobs that keep them indoors in harsh commercial lighting – this is often produced by white fluorescent tubes, which exclude some of the colours in the spectrum. If you must work inside, full-spectrum lights are healthier than fluorescent lights – they reduce irritability and promote productivity.

SAD season

The lack of sunlight during the long winter months changes the mood of most people. But for some, Seasonal Affective Disorder (or SAD) causes serious depression and low energy that only subside at the onset of spring. Women are more prone to SAD because of their complex hormonal makeup.

▾ *Our bodies have evolved over time to respond to the changing conditions of sunlight.*

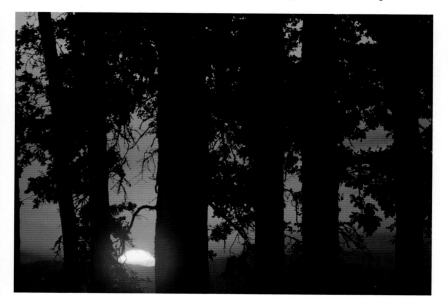

143 nurture optimism

The rumour is true: maintaining a positive outlook not only enhances but prolongs life and increases health. Septuagenarians all agree that looking on the bright side is one of the secrets of new youth.

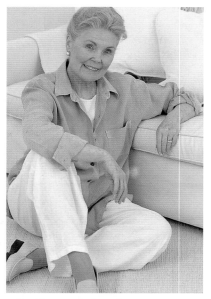

▲ *Look for ways to learn from every situation and you'll find satisfying solutions.*

Some people are more susceptible than others to slipping into negative thinking patterns – perhaps learned unconsciously from family, friends or the media. But by perpetuating a pessimistic outlook – such as always dwelling on what you lack – you may be wasting precious days and years

feeling irritated, dissatisfied and unhappy instead of savouring all the wonderful joys of life.

positive thinking

Fostering a sense of optimism for the present and future has huge benefits for psychological and physical health. Optimism can be enhanced by keeping busy – doing things that make you feel happy and enthused, setting new goals and meeting new people who encourage your positivity.

As we get older, a surplus of negative experiences – bad career moves, failed relationships, illness – may at times threaten to overwhelm us. You can move past these hardships by clearing your mind of emotional baggage from the past – visualize yourself throwing these "bags" away, leaving room for new experiences.

COUNT YOUR BLESSINGS
Begin the day in a positive frame of mind by making a list of five things for which you are grateful. As the days go by, you will see that you have more going for you than you realized.

144 life-affirming spirituality

You needn't be a member of an organized religion to explore your spirituality. Thinking about why you exist and what you are doing is an important part of living a long and meaningful life.

In today's materialistic Western society, it is sometimes easy to forget about the "invisible" life of the soul. When wrapped up in career, family and personal dramas or striving for material gains, you can forget that you are just one piece in a very vast puzzle. Taking time to reflect on your place in the universe can help you lead a more fulfilling life, whether you believe in a god or gods, or simply put your faith in the connections between people.

inner work

Scheduling time every day to think, meditate, pray or just "be" with yourself can help you live more comfortably with the changes that are inevitable for everyone. You may want to consider what happens after death, why events happen in the order that they do, why certain people have come into your life and what you can learn from them. Do you believe in free will or fate, or perhaps a combination of the two?

Knowing where you stand on these complex spiritual issues will help you make informed decisions; even though you may not have all the answers, at least you will be equipped with the tools to try and understand life more fully.

group spirituality

Many people find fulfilment by belonging to an organized faith that dictates a system of set principles and guidelines for living. Exploring the tenets of other faiths may help you to clarify your own views; you may also discover the positive similarities that exist between them all.

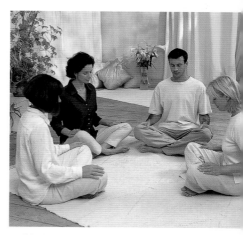

▲ Meditating with others can bring you closer to understanding the meaning of life.

145 creative fun

Having fun is a most underrated activity: from playfulness and fun have come some of the world's greatest inventions and works of art – as well as the most joyous personal pleasure.

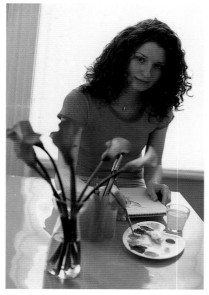

▲ *Relax and explore your creative side – the results might surprise you.*

Watch a child play with wooden blocks or let loose with finger paints – there's no doubt that having fun is directly linked with creativity. The greatest artists are daydreamers, so allow yourself to gaze into space; you may be surprised at what you can accomplish after a break from "reality".

explore strange new worlds

There is so much more to life than just your current situation – your home, work environment, city or village. By exploring different sides of yourself in a creative activity, you can expand your whole perspective of yourself and other people. The sense of accomplishment that comes from creating something from nothing may astound you – it will boost your confidence in all areas.

If you've always wanted to try pottery, cooking, saxophone–playing or creative writing, for example, now is the time to start. Find a course or other like-minded people who will learn to create with you, or get books and tapes and begin on your own.

don't be shy

Even if you think you won't become the greatest genius of all time in your chosen medium, don't let it stop you from beginning. Creativity is partly skill, partly unknown quantity – as any poet will tell you, there is a point when "something else" takes over and you're left with a little piece of magic to take back to the everyday world.

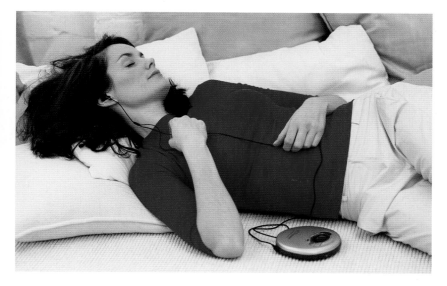

Don't allow yourself to be put off at your first attempt if you feel inadequate for the task. With a little practice you'll pick up skills that will soon become second nature, and before you know it you could become quite accomplished at your chosen activity.

revitalize your mind

Totally immersing yourself in an activity you really enjoy for a few hours a week can be enormously refreshing. It is an opportunity for your mind to concentrate on something totally, shutting out the realities and demands of modern living. The effect will be to exercise your mind in a different way, leaving it refreshed and revitalized and ready to take on your normal everyday activities with renewed vigour. Better still, break your usual routine with a holiday, if you can.

▲ ▼ Being immersed in a creative activity that you enjoy, whether it's a practical craft or listening to music, helps you to unwind.

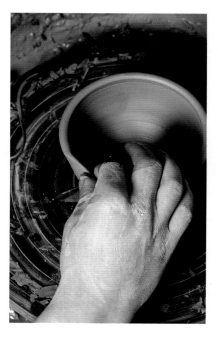

To give yourself a **rejuvenating** new look, experiment with clothes in **styles** and **colours** you wouldn't normally **choose**. Consign items you haven't worn for a **year** to a **charity shop**.

the effect of colour

Colour affects all levels of our being, and it is thought that our sensitivity to it has evolved as a response to the influence of sunlight. The fact that the warm colours of the spectrum – reds and oranges – activate and stimulate us, while the cool colours – blues and violets – calm us, probably derives from the biological triggers of daylight and nightfall.

clothes and colour

Whether we are aware of the process or not, we are all moved by colour, and it might explain why we like to wear certain colours at different times according to our mood or the impression we are trying to make.

Combinations of bright, festive colours are powerfully attractive, particularly to young children. For adults, who often wear more subtle shades or even monochrome colours, especially to work, the odd splash of colour in a tie, shirt, blouse or socks can make a huge statement about their personality or mood on that day.

black and white

Dark clothes can be worn to make the wearer inconspicuous, or they can make a bold statement of mystery and self control. They often say: "Notice my presence, but don't intrude into my space." White, on the other hand, can mean uncompromising clarity, but it can also take on a hint of other colour around it.

▼ *Below and left: The colours we choose to wear are an intensely personal choice .*

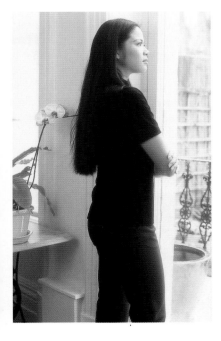
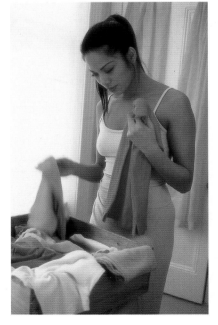

147 uplifting music therapy

There is nothing so moving as music – its effects on the body and soul vary endlessly, from encouraging healing feelings of catharsis to promoting a sense of ageless ecstasy.

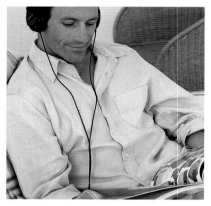

▲ *Music can recall people, times and places rather like an emotional history book.*

People use music every day as a therapy without even realizing it. When feeling melancholy, depressed or anxious, playing a recording of your favourite music lifts your mood instantly. Music can magnify positive emotions you are feeling as well; taking the journey from the first note of a song to the last is like an enjoyable workout for the psyche.

Playing a musical instrument exercises the brain and co-ordinates thought processes, helping to keep the mind sharp. With the pleasure and satisfaction that performing brings, comes a rush of endorphins, the brain's "feel-good" chemicals.

all together now

Drum circles, choir singing or playing instruments with a group can bring social, emotional and spiritual benefits – as well as increased physical health. Researchers have found that such activities strengthen the immune system; they raise levels of antibodies in the body, helping to fight disease.

Tibetan singing bowls offer music therapy even non-musicians can play. The tuned bowls are played by circling the rims with a mallet; the resulting sound fosters great mental focus.

▼ *The sound waves produced by Tibetan singing bowls create healing vibrations.*

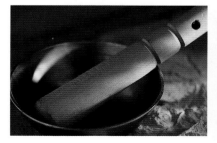

148 strengthening meditation

Anti-aging experts agree that meditation provides a sense of harmony that not only prolongs life, but improves its quality greatly. Here, visualizing a colour is used to balance the mind and emotions.

1 Slowly close your eyes and imagine yourself sitting in a green meadow near a cool, crystal-clear stream, with fragrant flowers surrounding you. The day is clear and bright, with a soft, gentle breeze swirling around you. The sky is blue with soft, white drifting clouds.

2 Choose a colour that you feel helps your sense of well-being. Look at one of the clouds above you, and let this cloud become suffused with your chosen colour. Watch it start to shimmer with its own sparkling light.

3 Allow the cloud to float over you; as it does, it releases a colourful shower of delicate, misty stars that sparkle all around your body and your being.

4 The mist settles on your skin, gently absorbing into your very core, completely saturating your system with its potent healing and strengthening vibrations.

5 Allow the colour to run through your body and your bloodstream for 3–4 minutes, soothing and restoring a sense of well-being. Feel the new pulse of energy in your cells.

6 Allow your pores to open and release the coloured vapour, taking any toxins or draining bad feelings with it. When the vapour runs clear, you can close your pores.

7 Sit quietly with your energized and balanced body for a few moments. Take three deep breaths, releasing each gently, before opening your eyes.

▼ *Regular meditation can bring an oasis of self-contained serenity to a hectic lifestyle.*

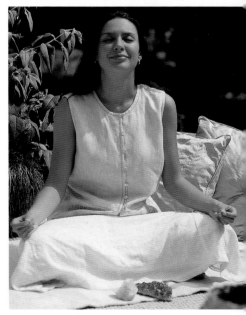

149 go wild

When you feel that life has become monotonous and you are stuck in a loop, trying something new and different will change your perspective, adding youthful excitement and sparkle.

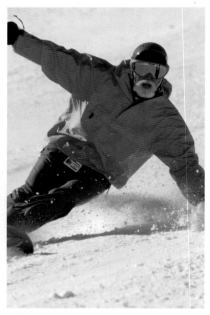

▲ *Bring new adventure to your life with a sport such as snowboarding or skiing.*

be a daredevil

If you are fit and eager, there is no reason not to try a new sport. Take up ice-skating, bowling, surfing, skiing – or if you enjoy an adrenaline thrill, extreme sports such as skydiving, hang-gliding or white water rafting.

In addition to being challenging and fun, they are a great way to meet new friends. Instruction is advised before beginning any of these activities.

Of course, you don't have to throw yourself down a mountain to go wild, you could sign up for tango lessons, dye your hair a different colour, paint your house pink or throw a large party – the possibilities are endless.

new sensations

Holidays are important, not only as a break from work, but as a refreshing change from normal routine. Visiting new places and cultures puts one's own life in perspective, and home tends to look more appealing on return. You may want to try a package holiday geared towards your interest, whether it's an art break in Paris or an African safari adventure.

If you are dissatisfied in your career, or just always wanted to learn about astrophysics, hairdressing, archeology or art, why not "go back to school"? It is never too late to explore new avenues and broaden your knowledge, for your career, or simply for your own interest.

150 essential relationships

People make the world go round – the longest and happiest lives are filled with friends and loved ones. Always make time for others, and you will share rewards that will delight and nurture your soul.

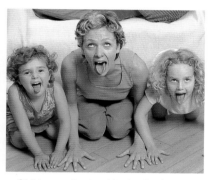

▲ Children understand fun instinctively, and the youngest adults never outgrow it.

different ages

Cultivate friendships with people of different ages and you will never want for new perspectives. Every age group has something to offer – from babies to great-grandads. Older people often bring surprising insights to situations and conversations; younger people have an optimism that is contagious – sharing their sense of hope can make life so much more enjoyable.

family life

Blood ties are among the closest relationships you will ever have, so it is a good idea to make the best of them

if you can. Your shared history with a favourite aunt, uncle, brother or sister who has known you since you were a baby can provide a sense of continuity that is unique. Staying close and providing mutual support lends you a confidence that will both help you weather life's storms and heighten its pleasures.

furry friends

Interacting with the animal kingdom – whether in nature or at home – is important for many people. Adopting a pet can add much joy and comfort to your life.

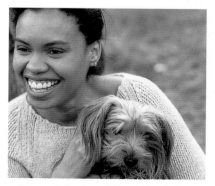

▲ Woman's (and man's) best friend: dogs repay human kindness many times over.

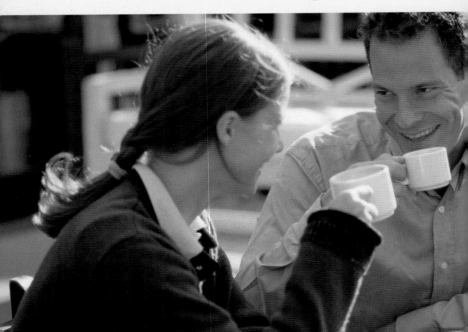

feeling se

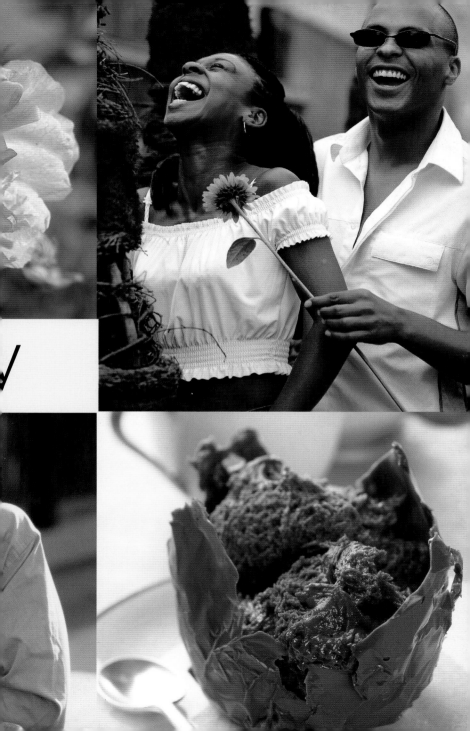

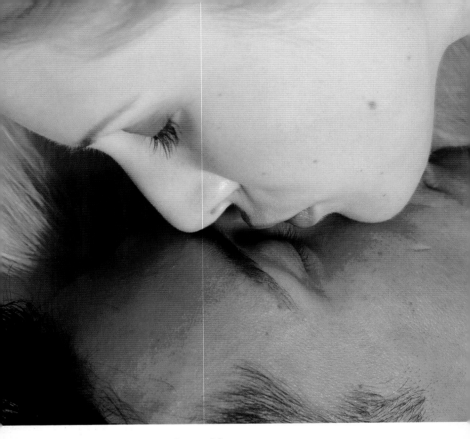

feeling sexy

We are sexual beings, and sexiness is thoroughly enmeshed with every aspect of our lives. Feeling sexy is all about feeling good about yourself, and this chapter suggests some simple ways to help you do that, with tips on using a range of complementary therapies and natural remedies.

You may feel that your general level of health is good, but a little extra effort can really supercharge your body. Stepping up the amount of exercise you do, and re-jigging your diet to include more high-energy foods, will quickly boost your metabolism, improving your cardio-vascular and respiratory health and balancing your hormones. Feeling fit and looking great is a real tonic for self-esteem, lifting the spirits and increasing zest for life.

When you're stressed, or depressed or tired, all kinds of pleasure can go out of the window. But a lack of sexual desire could also be induced by drugs. If you smoke, you're probably already familiar with all the good reasons why you need to give it up: the

◀ *Introducting seductive techniques, and playful, loving behaviour can kick start a sluggish sex life in a long-term relationhip*

effect on your sex life is just one of them. Smoking causes constriction of the blood vessels, and the consequent lowering of blood flow to the pelvic region leads to a decrease of sexual arousal in both men and women. Studies have found that in men between the ages of thirty and fifty, smoking increases the risk of impotence by fifty per cent.

Alcohol can also be a problem. Most drinkers would agree that a glass or two puts them in the mood for sex: they feel relaxed and shed any inhibitions. But heavy drinking has the opposite effect. Antidepressants, oral contraceptives and caffeine in coffee and fizzy drinks can also diminish your sex drive.

sex and sensuality

We talk about sexiness as a feeling, but rather than relaxing into that feeling we spend a great deal of time thinking about it instead. These days we are surrounded by images of sex: in films, on television, in magazines. Raunchy photographs and innuendo-laced slogans glare down from advertising hoardings, selling everything from cars to coffee. This kind of thing is part of the landscape and most people don't find it much of a thrill.

Good sex is about much more than the mechanics of coupling. It's about communication, confidence, a level of sensitivity and a sense of humour. Most of all it's about sensuality: the

engaging of all the senses to enable you to enjoy your own body and share that total enjoyment with your partner. There are plenty of ways to introduce more sensuality to your sex life. By concentrating on all five senses, you can find ways to make them all tingle with pleasure.

Be aware of the pressure of your touch when caressing your lover, from the gentlest brush of the fingertips to firmer strokes. Experience the feeling of different textures on your skin, such as the cool, slippery feel of silk or the

▾ *Take long hot baths with your partner, and unwind together after a stressful day.*

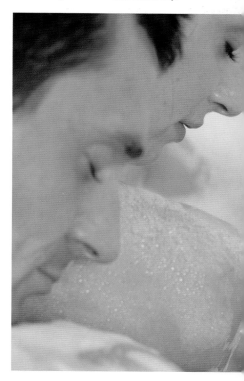

softness of velvet; play around with feathers, rubber, a soft brush.

Choose music to go with your mood. Mellow jazz or gentle classical music could help you unwind and relax. Brazilian or Cuban music is very sensual and can strongly influence the way you move together. Stimulate your sense of sight with atmospheric lighting such as candles or flickering firelight, creating an effect that flatters and pleases both of you. Explore all the contours of your bodies with your eyes, and watch your shadows moving on the wall.

The sense of smell has a powerful influence on your mood and emotions, and is especially important in the intimacy of lovemaking. The best smell is the smell of sex – that musky, heavy, natural perfume that attracts us to one another. But you can also rub musk or vanilla scented oil into your skin, perfume your hair, burn incense or light scented candles with sensuous aromas such as jasmine or sandalwood.

You'll be particularly sensitive to the taste of your bodies, but you might also enjoy some delicious morsels to tempt each other. Choose contrasting flavours and sensations: the satin smoothness of melting chocolate, the juicy tang of ripe mangoes, the salty slipperiness of oysters, the softness of cream, the sweet cold of ice cream.

This kind of delight in sensual pleasure isn't something to confine to sexual experience. A greater general sensual awareness can heighten your enjoyment of every daily activity, restoring your spirits and making you feel truly alive.

▾ *Sensual massage is an obvious start to sex, and can also be a good way to unwind.*

▸ *Make your evening routine something special with candlelight and wine.*

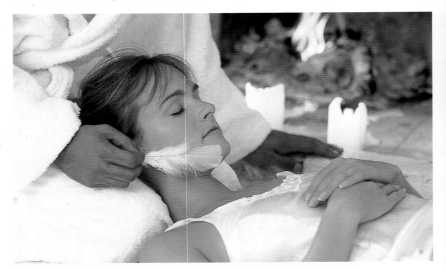

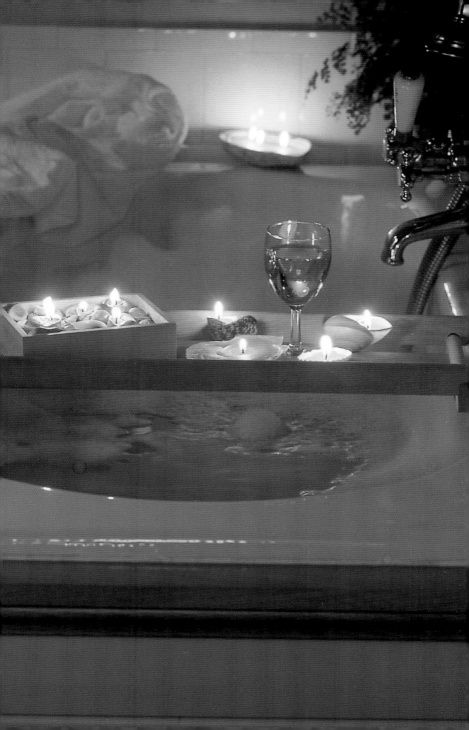

increasing
sexual desire

The quest for sure-fire aphrodisiacs is as old as humanity. Sexual desire is such a slippery commodity, and so important to our happiness, that every culture on earth seems to have developed its own repertoire of arousing foods, drinks and other remedies. Without making any claims for their efficacy, this chapter includes some of the most famous of these magic bullets – from oysters to chillies to the scent of jasmine. They might just work for you, and even if they don't they're fun to try.

The chapter also outlines a range of tried-and-tested natural therapies and remedies to tackle specific problems such as tiredness and stress, together with lots of delicious ideas to stimulate all your senses, from lighting your bedroom to scenting your bath. And finally, when you've made it to bed, there are some light-hearted suggestions for you and your lover to play around with. Sex is, after all, meant to be fun.

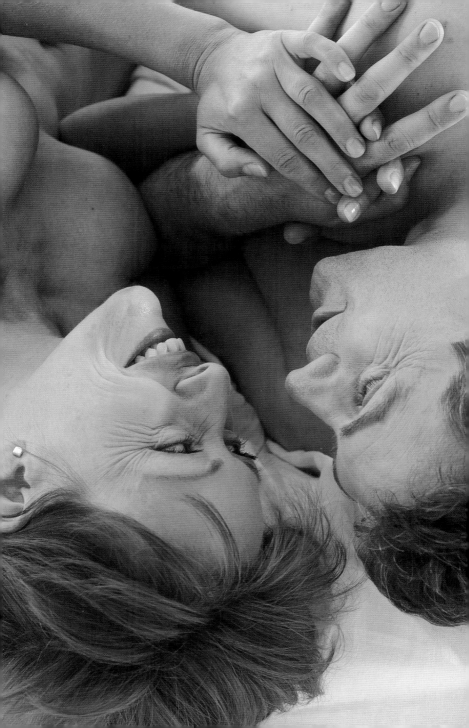

151 the game of seduction

It's often said that sex is ten per cent physical and ninety per cent emotional – the true foundations of sensuality, sexual enjoyment and fulfilment lie in the brain.

Unlike most animals, humans have sex for recreation, comfort and love, as well as for procreation. Preparation, anticipation and relaxation all start in the head: we need to be in the mood for sex, and this is controlled by the brain, the erotic epicentre of the body.

Dating, romancing, courting and flirting may seem a little old-fashioned to some people, but everyone is susceptible. Romance doesn't have to be flowers, toys and soppy letters. Small, thoughtful gestures usually have a far greater impact than large, lavish ones.

In the early stages of a relationship you can think of little else but each other and all your senses are alive with anticipation. The sky seems bluer, flowers smell sweeter and jokes seem funnier. Great memories are made during this period of getting to know one another, and can be evoked for ever after by a particular smell or a line of music. It is a sad fact that the better you get to know someone the more complacent you become about romance, but in a longstanding relationship it can still be disarming and delightful, and it is worth making the effort to revive it.

▾ *In the early stages of a relationship your focus on each other is strong and intense.*

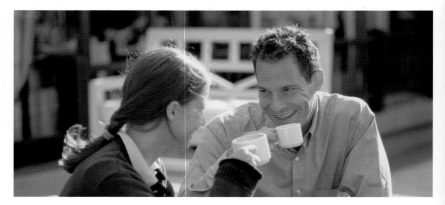

However long you've been in a relationship, **regular dating** keeps you feeling important to each other – remember how **excited** you felt the **first time** you went out together?

153 time together

However busy your lives, it's important to make time when your lives are not just running along parallel tracks. Take a walk with no fixed destination. Spend time together without pressure.

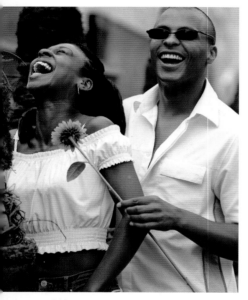

▲ Give your relationship the space it needs to be spontaneous and fun.

The ancient eastern philosophy of Tantra embraces sexuality as a means of reaching spiritual enlightenment, and cultivates the art of sex as a skilled spiritual practice. It sees sex as an expression of union, not just between you and your partner but with the whole of existence.

The pressures of modern life can leave you feeling isolated and unable to relate to each other or to experience each moment fully. Taking time out to renew your relationship with nature can help you feel that you are both part of the same whole and resolve that sense of separation.

at one with nature
Submerge yourselves in nature and renew your sense of wonder by making a serious commitment to break away from the daily responsibilities of work and home, and rediscover the magic of the natural world.

Lie on a beach on a warm moonlit night to gaze at the stars and listen to the roar of the waves. Walk through a forest and explore the myriad lives that coexist within it, or stroll across a soft carpet of meadow grass searching for wild flowers and becoming aware of the jubilant birdsong above you. Sit by a river and watch insects dance and buzz above the water. Feel yourselves to be part of the splendour of nature and carry this awareness into your love-making.

154 update your image

When you catch sight of yourself in a mirror you feel great if it gives you a buzz. If you've stopped noticing, it's time to splash out and make some changes – one change can lead to another.

It's said that beauty comes from within – and it does – but it can work the other way too. Knowing you look lovely puts a spring in your step, and its effect on your whole approach to life could surprise you.

Advertisers promise "a whole new you" with every new beauty product: the fashion and beauty industries are founded on our insecurities about our appearance, and both men and women are susceptible. A makeover won't transform your life, but it can be a great morale-boost, helping you see yourself as the sexy person you are.

Most people wear their hair the same way for years without changing it. A change of style can be a real tonic. You'll get noticed and complimented – with luck by your partner, but certainly by everyone else. Consider changing the colour too. It's amazing what a difference even the softest tint can make to your hair, your face and your overall image.

When you shop for clothes, dare to try on colours and styles you wouldn't normally choose. And buying sexy underwear might seem like a cliché, but it works.

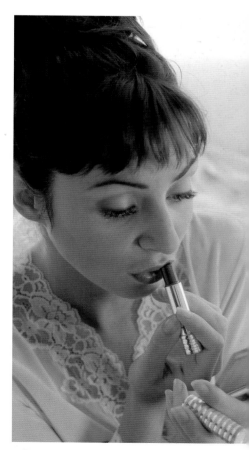

▲ *Devote some time to a bit of preening, it will boost your self-esteem amazingly.*

155 stress-busting exercise

Great sex goes with good health, and an important aspect of keeping well is keeping fit. Regular exercise will not only keep your body in shape but will reduce stress and make you happier.

Jogging, swimming, cycling and walking are all excellent aerobic sports. The most important thing is to choose a form of exercise that you enjoy so that it's no problem finding time for regular sessions – there's no point in joining a gym if you stop going after a few weeks. Don't overdo things, but start gently and gradually build up your stamina, strength and suppleness. Try to make some exercise a part of your daily routine, even if it's just a brisk walk on your way to work.

Exercise is just as important when you're young as when you are older, and you benefit by keeping your heart and lungs strong and your muscles toned. Aerobic exercise burns fat, boosts the immune system, aids flexibility and improves sleep, making you feel healthier, livelier and sexier.

freeing the mind

As well as toning your body, exercise is good for your mind. It's a great stress-reliever, distracting you from nagging anxieties and, by releasing tension in your body, helping to free up your mind too. Vigorous activity causes a rise in the level of endorphins in the blood and these substances, the body's natural painkillers, are thought to be connected with feelings of euphoria and the release of sex hormones. (Endorphins are also produced during sex.) The sense of achievement you get after exercise will raise self-esteem, you'll feel proud of your fitter body – and happy to show it off.

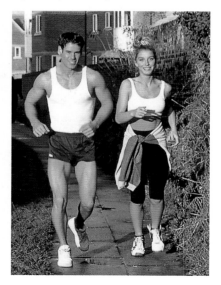

◄ *Exercising together is a great way to create a bond while improving fitness.*

156 tension-relieving stretches

This simple sequence of stretching exercises helps to release tension in the spine and tones all the organs in the pelvic basin, as well as improving blood flow to and from the area.

1 For twisting sit-ups, lie on your back with your legs bent, feet apart, and hands behind your head. Breathe in, then, as you exhale, raise your head and one shoulder, at the same time raising your leg so that opposite elbow and knee approach each other. Lower your shoulder and knee, then repeat on the other side.

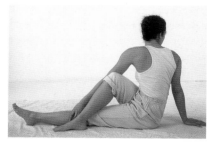

2 Sitting with your legs straight out in front of you, bend one leg and place the foot on the outside of the other leg. Reach around the bent leg with the opposite arm to hold the straight leg and twist your upper body. Relax and repeat on the other side.

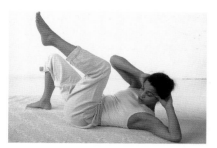

3 Bend both legs and bring the soles of the feet together. Clasp the feet with your hands and try to pull them a little closer to your body. Let the knees drop towards the floor. Hold the stretch, relax and repeat.

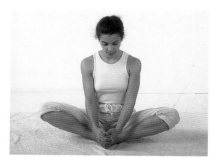

157 sexercises

Like any other muscles, the pelvic floor muscles need to be kept toned. Apart from enhancing your sex life, a strong pelvic floor avoids problems with bladder and bowel control in later life.

The pubcoccygeus (PC) muscle resembles a hammock slung between the legs, and is the one that contracts at a rate of just under once a second during orgasm. It tends to become flabbier with age, and other factors – childbirth, weight gain or a chronic cough – can weaken it further.

for her

Exercises designed to strengthen the pelvic muscles and tighten the vagina were practised by women in ancient China and India. Kegel exercises, which are now widely used, were devised by Dr Arnold Kegel in 1948 as a means of reducing incontinence after childbirth, but they can also help intensify and prolong orgasms.

You first need to locate and isolate the correct muscle, and the easiest way to do this is to stop and start the flow while urinating (although you should not do Kegel exercises during urination). Exercise by tightening and relaxing the muscle twenty times in a session and build up to sixty or more. Then prolong each squeeze to five seconds. You can do them anywhere: on a train, in the office, or in bed.

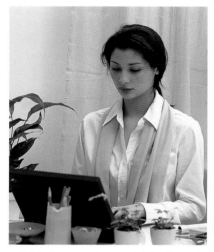

▲ Pelvic floor exercises are totally discreet, can be done almost anywhere.

for him

Kegel exercises are also suitable for men. An additional exercise is to place a small damp towel on your erect penis and practise moving it up and down. Strong pelvic floor muscles give you greater control over the timing of your orgasm, and a recent study of older men has shown that pelvic floor exercises can help to restore erectile function.

158 mind-clearing meditation

Meditation can transform your life and give you the time and space to explore different aspects of yourself and your relationship. You can practise alone or with your partner.

Meditation is a way of focusing the mind and stilling the mental chatter that distracts us from concentrated attention. Even while we're enjoying something, we're only half there, with part of our mind wandering along other tracks. Meditating helps us to live in the moment.

alpha waves
Each time you meditate, your heart slows, your blood pressure drops and your brain starts to produce alpha waves. You may have experienced the alpha state by chance when you were very relaxed. When you slip into it you feel a sense of deep contentment. Niggling worries vanish. Meditation is a simple technique for finding that calm space whenever you need it.

learning to meditate
It's easiest to get into the meditation habit if you do it at the same time and place every day. It doesn't have to take long: set a timer for ten minutes once a day. The simplest way to start is to count your breaths. Sit comfortably with your back straight and let your breathing slow down, then count the length of each breath just before you take a new one. Count up to ten, then start again. Keep your attention on your breathing. Note how the air feels as it enters and leaves your body. As thoughts enter your mind, let them drift away. Before long it becomes easier to bring your focus back after each detour. You stop fidgeting and begin to feel a sense of peace.

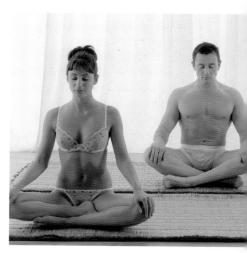

▸ *Try a joint meditation session as a prelude to making love.*

159 boost your confidence

Don't wait to hear compliments from others: just tell yourself you're great. Emphasize all your positive attributes and you'll see what an attractive and irresistible person you really are.

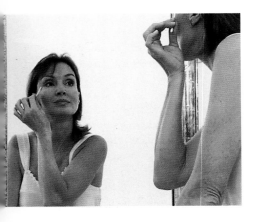

◄ Build your affirmations into your usual morning or evening routines.

Lack of confidence can dull your sexual energy and enjoyment just as it limits your potential in other aspects of life. Feeling really good about yourself has the opposite effect. If you are a severe self-critic you already know how influential your own voice is, because you believe it. You can use its power to emphasize your positive aspects instead. Making affirmations during meditation is a deceptively simple but effective device that can change the way you think about yourself and the way you act.

The technique requires you to say out loud, positive statements about

yourself as you wish to be. Be aware of any negative statements you habitually make, such as "I find it hard to talk to people," or "I am too fat". You are reinforcing these self-limiting beliefs each time they slip into your conversation, but you can use affirmations to change such beliefs. The affirmations should be in the present tense and should be positively phrased.

- I like my... [eyes/hair/legs...]
- I am proud of my... [intelligence/sense of humour/achievement]
- My friendship is valuable to... [name of person]
- I am lovable and can give love.

Keeping the statements short will give them more impact. You don't have to believe them at first, but if you repeat them often enough, they start to make a difference. Belief will come and your feeling of self-worth will grow.

160 sleep strategies

Feeling too tired to make love at the end of the day is a common problem. Stress and overwork can cause a loss of libido and can also result in insomnia, creating a vicious cycle of tiredness.

▸ *Making sure you both get enough sleep will improve your energy levels in all areas.*

To break the stress cycle, learning to relax needs to be built into a daily pattern that also makes time for healthy meals and some regular exercise. It may be that only one of you is having disturbed nights, but relaxing rituals that prepare you for sleep are a pleasure to share.

Make your bedroom as calm and serene as possible, banning the television, computers and work-related clutter to create a peaceful, secure cocoon. Avoid eating late at night, and instead of tea or coffee try a relaxing herbal infusion. Unwind in a warm bath – together if you like – scented with a blend of sedative essential oils such as rose, lavender and ylang ylang. Read a novel or listen to gentle music to take your mind off the concerns of the day before you settle down and try to sleep.

If you do wake during the night, don't just lie there allowing yourself to get tense and panicky. If a heavy workload is causing stress, one way to free your mind at night is to write

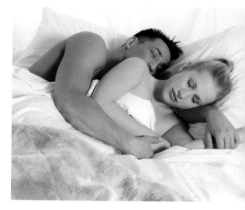

down a list of all the tasks you need to do tomorrow so that you can stop running through them in your head.

post-coital sleep
Of course, sex itself can be an effective aid to falling asleep – particularly for men. If you are a woman who enjoys that precious relaxed time of lying together, having a partner who falls instantly asleep can be exasperating. On the other hand, you could choose to see it as an indication of his total security and trust in you, and just enjoy lying next to him in a warm glow until you drift off to sleep too.

161 supple sensuality

Yoga works to integrate mind, body and spirit. The regular postures of hatha yoga can help you to relax or feel more energetic. For a surge of energy work through dynamic poses such as the Warrior.

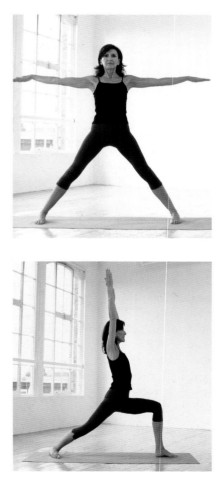

1 Stand with feet together and arms at your side, inhale deeply, and jump or step the feet 1–1.2m/3–4ft apart, and raise the arms to shoulder level. Turn the palms upwards and extend the arms towards the ceiling, keeping the elbows straight and the palms facing one another. Turn the right foot and leg in deeply, about 40 degrees, and the left foot out 90 degrees. At the same time, turn the hips, trunk and shoulders to the left. Both sides of the trunk should be parallel – so bring the right hip forwards, while taking the left hip slightly back, to keep them even.

2 Exhale and bend the left leg to form a 90-degree angle. Extend the trunk upwards, as if it were being lifted out of the hips. Move the shoulder blades into the body to open the chest. Extend the chin towards the ceiling and look up. Maintain the full extension on the back leg and keep the hips, shoulders and trunk rotating to the left. Hold for 20–30 seconds, inhale, come up and lower the arms. Repeat on the other side, coming back to the original position, facing forwards with feet together and arms by the side .

162 dynamic breath

Breathing exercises, or pranayama, are an essential aspect of yoga. The breath is considered to carry prana, the life force, around the body to revitalize the entire being.

Our breathing patterns reflect our emotional and mental state. When we are nervous or strained, our breathing tends to be shallow and fast. Taking control of this, and slowing down the breathing calms the nervous system and dissolves stress. Be aware of how you are breathing during the day, and when the rate increases, consciously bring it down to a slower speed. Then try either of these two breathing exercises to revitalize your life force.

alternate nostril breathing

1 Sitting erect, place your right hand against your face. Your eyes may be closed, or open and gazing softly ahead. Close your right nostril with your thumb and breathe in through the left nostril.

2 Release the right nostril and close the left. Breathe out slowly, then in again, through your right nostril. Then open the left nostril, close the right and breathe out. Repeat the sequence five times.

▶ *Breathing exercises just need a few moments of quiet.*

bee breath

This is a relaxing technique that relieves insomnia and produces a meditative state. It can also give you a deliciously sexy voice, as it releases tension in the throat.

1 Sit upright with your eyes closed. Take a long breath in, then breathe out slowly through your nose, making a continuous humming noise.

2 Relax and let the sound become deep and rich. Repeat five times, focusing your mind on the sound.

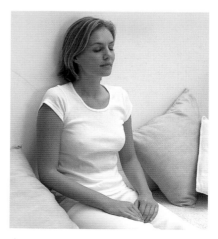

163 herbs to give you a lift

When your libido needs a boost, try a herbal tea. Among medicinal herbs there are several with ancient reputations as aphrodisiacs. They work by invigorating and nourishing the nervous system.

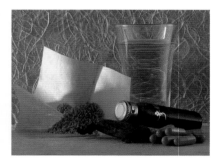

korean ginseng (*panax sp.*)
Ginseng — whose name means "wonder of the world" – spurs energy of every kind and increases strength and stamina. By improving the production of adrenal hormones, it helps the body to adapt to stress and fights fatigue. But it should be taken only as a short-term remedy (not more than six weeks).

> **ENERGIZING TEA**
> Put 1 tsp dried damiana and 1 tsp dried vervain in a pot and pour on 600ml/1 pint/2 ½ cups boiling water. Steep for 10 minutes then strain and flavour with ginger or honey. Drink two cups a day.

◀ *Consulting a herbalist is a good way of making sure you get the right remedy.*

damiana (*turnera diffusa*)
This Central American herb is a traditional remedy for reviving sexual function (it was previously called Turnera aphrodisiaca) as it stimulates the reproductive organs and boosts blood flow. It works as a tonic for both the nervous and hormonal systems,

vervain (*verbena officinalis*)
The Romans considered vervain a magical herb and used it to alleviate depression and nervous exhaustion as well as for its aphrodisiac potency. It has a slightly sedative effect, releasing tension and stress.

wild oats (*avena sativa*)
Oats are an excellent general tonic – they'll give you energy and lift your mood. They're also a good source of vitamin E, iron, zinc, manganese and protein. A traditional breakfast of porridge every morning is a great idea, but there are lots of other delicious ways to eat oats, such as flapjacks and oatcakes.

164 help from homeopathy

Feeling sexually fulfilled is a matter of the mind and emotions as much as physical responses, so if you're having problems with a low sex drive homeopathy might help.

Many people respond positively to homeopathy, which is based on the premise that "like cures like". The remedies are extremely dilute forms of substances that in their normal form would cause the symptoms presented. They're completely safe. Homeopaths treat a person as a whole, not as a list of symptoms, taking into account your character, lifestyle, habits, medical history, and the relationships between all aspects of your life. The prescription is likely to be different in every case, but one of the following remedies might be used for sexual problems.

Agnus castus: for impotence or failure to reach orgasm through fatigue and lack of energy.

Graphites: for men with a positive aversion to sex.

Lycopodium: to help in premature ejaculation or lack of erection.

Sepia: for women who feel irritable, exhausted and indifferent to sex.

Natrum mur: for women who are suffering a loss of libido associated with grief, and who are unable to let go of their emotions.

▼ *The distinctive, tiny homeopathic pills are much easier to take than other medicine.*

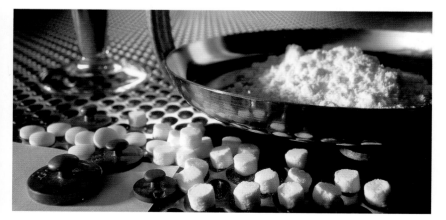

flower essences for fun

Sex is bound to be more fun when you're feeling sunny and optimistic. Bach flower remedies harness the natural energy of plants to balance your emotions and cheer you up.

You can swallow a few drops of any or all of the following essences each day to keep your spirits high, and there are other ways in which you and your partner can share their effects. Just add a few drops to a water spray and spritz the bedroom, not forgetting the bed, or add them to a scented bath oil. When you wash clothes and bedlinen, add flower essences to the final rinse.

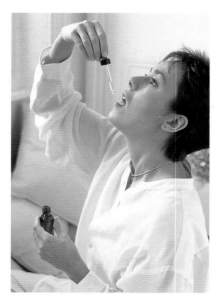

borage
If you're sad, borage cheers you up and makes you feel buoyant and bold.

daffodil
When your ego needs a boost, daffodil essence removes self-doubt and helps you appreciate your own talents, so that life can blossom again.

zinnia
This essence is for people who are taking life too seriously; it restores spontaneity and playfulness and helps you take a detached view – and have a laugh at yourself.

dandelion
Try dandelion when you've too much to do and you're feeling stressed. It will help you relax and give you a feeling of effortless energy.

buttercup
Good for a lack of self-esteem, buttercup warms and nourishes the being with golden light.

◀ *Bach remedies are a gentle and effective way of treating emotional problems.*

crystal energy focus

Gemstones have long been recognized as possessing healing properties. Experimenting with different crystals may help you find the one that has a particular resonance for you.

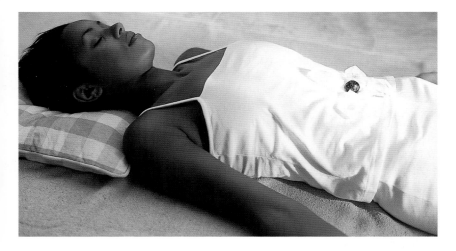

The red garnet is the finest energizing stone for the body, especially when it's cut. The facets increase the liveliness of the stone and act like a lens, focusing light with more intensity. Fiery garnet can be placed wherever you feel a lack of energy. It acts as a "starter motor" and very often needs only a short while to do its work.

a balancing placement

After a hard day's work it can sometimes take a long time to "wind down" and feel relaxed enough to

▲ *Lying for a few minutes with a red garnet placement will help increase your energy.*

enjoy yourself. A simple placement of stones can help you to feel calm and refreshed after a couple of minutes.

Lying down comfortably, place a garnet at the centre of the body and surround it with four clear quartz cyrstals, points facing outwards. The quartz will help increase the garnet's energy and distribute it. Lie in this position for 4–5 minutes, then remove the stones.

167 reflexology energizer

After a reflexology session, most people are deeply relaxed, but soon begin to feel energized and motivated. This is an intimate, caring touch therapy that can awaken your senses.

A foot massage, working on reflexology principles, is a gentle way of establishing touch between you both. For a more vigorous and thorough reflexology session, consult a practitioner.

CAUTION
If you choose to try reflexology on your partner, it is important that he or she is in good health.

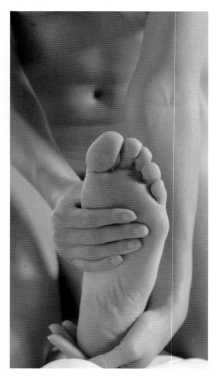

stimulating the body's systems
1 Massage the whole of the feet vigorously to get the circulation going.

2 Applying downward pressure with the tip of the thumb, "thumbwalk" along the instep to stimulate the nervous system in the spinal cord.

3 Work the ball of the foot, corresponding to the chest, to establish regular, deep breathing.

4 Work the pituitary reflex in the centre of the big toe-print: this is the master gland, which controls the other endocrine glands and produces hormones involved in many bodily systems, including sexual functioning.

◄ *You can perform this quick foot massage on yourself or on your partner.*

168 high-energy eating

Boost your sexual energy, as well as your general health, by sticking to a super-nourishing diet rich in fresh, natural foods. Cut down on sugar-rich and salty snacks.

A diet that makes you feel more energetic is based on natural, nutritious, wholesome ingredients, rather than fatty fast foods. To boost your energy levels, snack on fresh and dried fruits that are high in natural sugars, such as pears, kiwi fruit and apricots. Eat plenty of vegetables such as peas, spinach, cabbage and onions.

VITAL VITAMINS AND MINERALS

A well-balanced diet will contain all the vitamins and minerals you need for a healthy libido, including the following:

Vitamin E: protects blood cells and tissues, and may have a direct effect on fertility and sexual function.

Vitamin B3/niacin: acts as a vasodilator, increasing blood flow to the skin.

Vitamin B8/folic acid: assists ovarian function and sperm production.

Zinc: thought to support male prostate function, sperm count and libido.

Selenium: may stimulate sexual energy.

Iodine: supports the thyroid gland, improves desire and capacity.

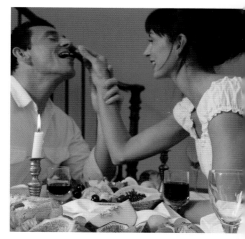

▲ Food can be fun as well as healthy, choose exotic fruit to share together.

Include oily fish, such as salmon and mackerel, poultry and lean red meat such as game and lean beef.

Nuts, brown rice, seeds, pulses and whole grains are packed with energy-giving protein and carbohydrates, they are also rich in valuable minerals and vitamins. Use cold-pressed oils such as olive, grapeseed or sunflower with salads. Don't skip dairy foods but stick to skimmed or semi-skimmed milk and natural low-fat yogurt.

169 erotic feasts

Like great sex, the enjoyment of fantastic food with your partner can be a sublime experience that stimulates all the senses. It makes perfect sense to put the two together.

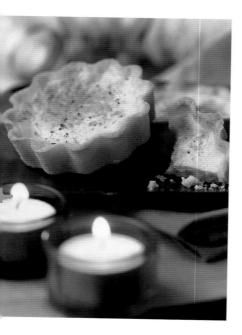

◀ *Small amounts of intensely sweet food will give you a sudden energy burst.*

Choose lovely sensual food, with buttery sauces to glisten alluringly on your lips and titbits that you can proffer to your partner across a candlelit table.

If the prospect of making love wipes away your appetite beforehand, eating after sex can be divine. Sharing food in bed creates a playful, happy atmosphere, and might even give you the energy to start all over again. You can go and raid the fridge together (which you'll have carefully pre-stocked with delicious treats like sushi, mangoes, strawberries and ice cream).

a midnight feast

Prepare a perfect treat – oysters and champagne, say – but hide it from your partner. Have a normal evening with a light meal, then say you're tired and go to bed early. Once your partner's asleep you can sneak out of bed, set the scene with candles and soft music and retrieve the feast from the kitchen. Wake your partner gently and enjoy a night of passion.

Preparing a special meal for your lover is a time-honoured seduction technique. Gazing across the table as you peel a prawn or sink your teeth into a ripe fig can make you both tingle with anticipation. If you're choosing a menu with seduction in mind, keep it light – you don't want to end up full and slumped on the sofa.

170 exotics & curiosities

Is there really such a thing as an aphrodisiac? In every culture, particular delicacies are credited with the ability to drive women mad with passion or give men the stamina to make love all weekend.

Aphrodisiacs are named after the Greek goddess of love, Aphrodite, but the idea is a universal one. Hopeful lovers have enlisted the help of foods and potions of all descriptions, from chocolate to powdered rhino horn.

Rare and exotic foods, particularly, are believed to have this special power. The more outlandish and expensive they are, the better they work – and perhaps there's some truth in this. You may want your lover to realize that you are using an aphrodisiac to seduce him or her, and this could be quite persuasive in itself.

truffles

In one study, women who were shown photographs of men thought they looked sexier when the smell of truffles was wafted past them. To test the effect for yourself, try shavings of fresh black or white truffle scattered over scrambled eggs or fresh pasta.

caviar

The ultimate luxury food: eating it is certainly a sensual experience. It's also rich in zinc, so it could really be good for the male libido.

fugu

The Japanese puffer fish is potentially deadly if not properly prepared, yet it's a costly and much sought-after delicacy. Japanese men take an aphrodisiac potion made by mixing its sperm with hot sake.

snake blood

In parts of Asia it's believed that blood freshly pumped from a dying snake - preferably poisonous – is a potent aphrodisiac. Some bars serve vodka and blood cocktails.

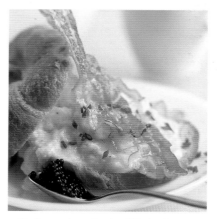

▲ *Caviar can be eaten in all kinds of ways and with almost any meal.*

171 seductive salads

Plenty of raw food in your diet keeps all the body's systems working at full power, but some salad ingredients just seem to have the edge when it comes to sex.

All fresh, "live" raw vegetables and fruits contain vital enzymes – destroyed by cooking – that enhance digestion and have a great de-toxing effect. Big bowls of exciting salads will keep your skin glowing and your eyes bright, and help you stay lean and

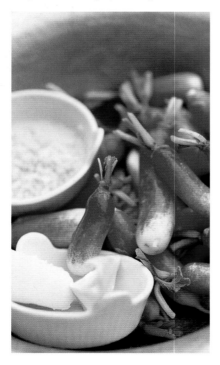

lively. For extra sex appeal, try some of these foods, all of which have an overt or more subtle sexual reputation.

When they first reached Europe from South America, tomatoes were known as "love apples". This may have been due to a simple mistranslation, but the link endured, helped by their voluptuous form and colour.

The Aztec name for the avocado means "testicle tree", and their shape, hanging in pairs on the branch, is unmistakably suggestive, leading to their reputation as a powerful aphrodisiac. Young girls were forbidden to pick them. The flesh is luscious and has a sensuous texture.

Sweet basil is said to stimulate sex drive and instil a sense of wellbeing.

Radishes were valued as a divine aphrodisiac by the ancient Egyptians, perhaps because their peppery flavour tickled the palate, or perhaps because of their colour and shape.

Fennel is regarded as a sexual stimulant in India, as it was by the ancient Greeks.

◄ *Dipping radishes in soft butter and then salt is a traditional French hors d'oeuvres.*

172 asparagus to share

There's no denying the phallic connotations of asparagus. For a delicious, sensuous experience, feed your lover the tender spears, with melted butter or the unctuous dressing in this recipe.

It's said that you should eat asparagus for three days for the most powerful effect – why not try it during its brief in-season period, when there is plenty of it about?

asparagus with creamy raspberry vinaigrette
350g/¾lb asparagus spears
15ml/1 tbsp raspberry vinegar
2.5ml/½ tsp Dijon mustard
45ml/3 tbsp sunflower oil
15ml/1 tsp soured cream
salt and white pepper
a few fresh raspberries

1 Fill a wide pan with water and bring to the boil. Trim the ends of the asparagus spears. Lower into the water and cook for 2 minutes or until just tender. Remove with a slotted spoon and drain. Leave to cool while you make the dressing.

2 Blend the vinegar with the mustard then gradually stir in the oil. Add the soured cream and season to taste.

3 Drizzle the dressing over the asparagus and serve with raspberries.

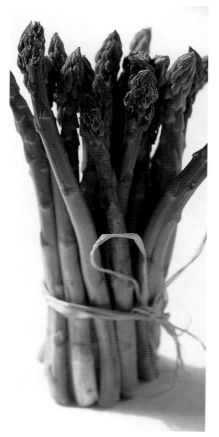

▲ *Use the young slender spears for the tenderest taste experience.*

173 luxurious seafood

A seafood feast is a fantastic start to a night of hedonistic pleasure. Choose lobster for sheer indulgence, or go for the classic seductive combination of oysters and champagne.

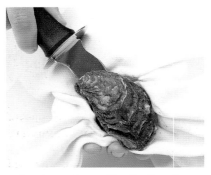

▲ *Opening oysters and feeding them to your partner can make an entire love feast.*

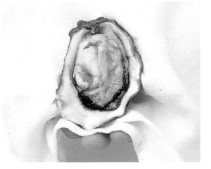

▲ *Oysters not only feel sensuous, but they have an undeniably sexy appearance.*

Fish of all kinds rightly claim a place on the list of aphrodisiacs – Aphrodite did, after all, emerge from the sea. They're also very nutritious, high in protein to keep up your stamina, zinc to increase testosterone levels, and Omega-3 fatty acids for circulation.

Apart from being a luxurious treat, oysters are the ultimate in sensual eating. Soft and wet, they slip smoothly down the throat, and their little folds and fissures give them an unmistakable resemblance to female genitalia. Made for feeding to each other: an oyster feast is the perfect party for two.

buying and preparing oysters

Make sure the shells are firmly shut when you buy oysters. Scrub the shells and keep them flat-side up to retain all the juices. Keep them cool, and eat them on the same day.

To open an oyster, grasp it firmly in a cloth with the hinge towards you. Press the point of the oyster knife into the hinge and rotate it to dislodge the upper shell. Slide the blade over the meat to sever the upper muscle. Do the same under the meat to free the oyster. Remove any fragments of shell and eat with lemon juice, black pepper and a drop of Tabasco.

174 nuts & honey

Drizzle honey over Greek yogurt and scatter it liberally with nuts and you'll be benefiting from two ancient sex secrets of the Mediterranean. It'll also make a delicious start to breakfast in bed.

For centuries, nuts have been mixed with honey for love potions. The Arabic sex manual, *The Perfumed Garden,* recommends a glass of thick honey, twenty almonds and a hundred pine nuts, repeated for three nights, to restore a man's sexual vigour.

Pine nuts are widely regarded as an aphrodisiac, and they are in fact a good source of zinc, which is said to boost the sex drive by raising

RUNNY HONEY
Drizzle a trail over your partner's body that you can then lick off – or plot a path over yourself and lead your lover in any direction you want.

testosterone levels. So serve lashings of fresh pesto with pasta, or toast the nuts and scatter them over salads.

The smell of almonds is supposed to induce passion in women, and they have long been a symbol of fertility, as are walnuts (which the Romans threw at newlyweds). All kinds of nuts are good energy foods.

honey

The Egyptians used honey as a cure for most things, including impotence. The honeymoon gets its name from the time when couples were encouraged to drink mead – made from fermented honey – to keep them going. Honey is high in B vitamins and amino acids which keep the body performing at its peak.

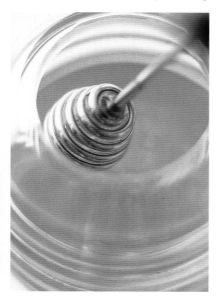

◄ *Honey has been given all kinds of medical and mystical properties through the ages.*

175 turning up the heat

Spicy foods are viewed as aphrodisiacs because their effects on the body – raising the heart rate and making you sweat – are similar to some of the reactions experienced during sex.

Though not necessarily hot, Indian cooking is distinctively spicy and is characterized by the use of a greater range of dried spices than any other cuisine. Up to fifteen spices may be blended to flavour one dish. India is a vast country and the style of cooking varies enormously from region to region, but the spices most often used include coriander, cumin, turmeric, black pepper, mustard seeds, fennel seeds, cardamom, cloves, garlic and ginger. Chillies are valued for both fire and flavour; some Indians dishes are extremely hot, but in others spices are used with rare subtlety.

Chinese cooks use liberal amounts of fresh ginger and garlic. They favour spices such as sesame seeds and star anise, the predominant flavour of their five spice blend. The spices of this blend are finely ground to quickly release their flavour in stir-fries.

Thai dishes tend to be very hot, with the tiny – and fiery – Thai chillies appearing in many dishes. The heat, however, is tempered by the fresh light flavours of lemon grass and kaffir lime leaves and the soothing effect of coconut milk.

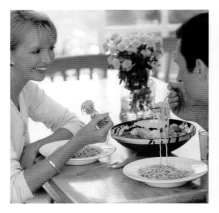

▲ Dishes full of tantalizing flavours are great to share.

Thai green chicken curry
450ml/¾ pint/2 cups chicken stock
2 boneless, skinless chicken breasts, sliced into strips
200ml/7fl oz can coconut milk
30ml/2 tbsp chopped fresh coriander (cilantro)
shredded spring onions (scallions) and shredded red (bell) pepper, to serve

▸ Whether or not chillies lift your libido, this Thai curry is a wonderfully warming dish.

for the green curry paste:
5 fresh green chillies, chopped
6 shallots, chopped
3 garlic cloves
75g/3oz fresh coriander (cilantro)
finely grated rind of 1 lime
5ml/1 tsp dried shrimp paste
small piece of fresh root ginger, chopped
1 small stick lemon grass, chopped
2.5ml/½ tsp ground turmeric
2.5ml/½ tsp ground cumin
10ml/2 tsp ground coriander
30ml/2 tbsp vegetable oil
salt and ground black pepper

1 Process the green curry paste ingredients until smooth. Whisk a little of the stock with half the paste in a frying pan (the rest will keep, refrigerated, for about a month). Bring to the boil and simmer for about 2 minutes until the liquid has evaporated.

2 Add the chicken and remaining stock and stir. Bring to the boil and simmer for 10 minutes. Stir in the coconut milk and simmer for 5 minutes.

3 Add the coriander and season to taste. Serve sprinkled with shredded spring onions and red pepper.

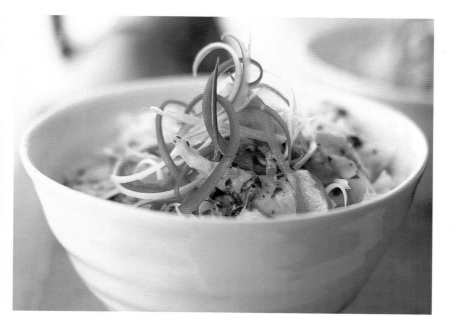

176 irresistible chocolate

Any erotic feast has to include a liberal supply of chocolate. It's said that chocolate contains a natural substance that causes the same physical reaction as falling in love.

Casanova described hot chocolate as "the elixir of love" and drank it instead of champagne. Chocolate's reputation for stimulating sexual desire came to Europe with the Spanish conquistadors, and whether or not it's true, the idea has been firmly fixed ever since. Modern adverts, particularly those aimed at women, are heavy with innuendo associating chocolate with indulgent passion. Dark chocolate, particularly, is clearly associated with wicked pleasures.

One of the reasons we love chocolate so much is the pure physical pleasure we get from the whole experience of eating it: not just its taste, but its heavy perfume and smooth, melting texture. The flavour of chocolate — two and a half times more complex than any other food — overwhelms the tastebuds, just as good sex overwhelms the body.

So chocolate's X-rated character makes it a winner in love-making. Simply melted by itself, or turned into a velvety mousse or a glistening sauce, it will trail beguilingly over warm skin, wherever you'd most enjoy having it licked off.

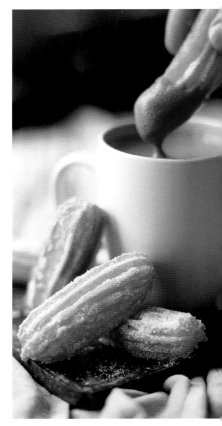

▲ Drink thick hot chocolate in bed together, morning or night, and dip crisp, warm churros into it for a powerful energy surge.

chocolate and espresso mousse

Heady, aromatic espresso coffee adds a distinctive flavour to this smooth, rich mousse. The stylish chocolate cups make this a truly sensual treat but can be omitted if you are worried about your waistline. Makes four servings.

225g/8oz plain (semisweet)
    chocolate
45ml/3 tbsp brewed espresso
25g/1oz/2 tbsp unsalted butter
4 eggs, separated
sprigs of fresh mint, to decorate
    (optional)
mascarpone or clotted cream, to serve
    (optional)
for the chocolate cups 225g/8oz
    plain (semisweet) chocolate

1 For each chocolate cup, cut a double thickness 15cm/6in square of foil. Mould it around a small orange, leaving the edges and corners loose to make a cup shape. Remove the orange and press the bottom of the foil case gently on a work surface to make a flat base.

2 Break the plain chocolate into small pieces and place in a bowl set over a pan of very hot water. Stir occasionally until the chocolate has melted.

3 Spoon the chocolate into the foil cups, spreading it up the sides with the back of a spoon to give a ragged edge. Refrigerate for 30 minutes.

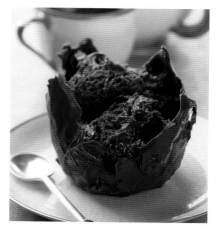

▲ This rich, smooth dessert is the perfect conclusion to a romantic dinner.

4 Gently peel away the foil, starting at the top edge.

5 To make the chocolate mousse, put the plain chocolate and espresso into a bowl set over a pan of hot water and allow to melt as before. When it is smooth and liquid, add the unsalted butter, a little at a time. Remove the pan from the heat then gently stir in the egg yolks.

6 Whisk the egg whites in a bowl until stiff, but not dry, then fold them into the chocolate mixture. Pour into a bowl and refrigerate for at least 3 hours.

7 To serve, scoop the chilled mousse into the chocolate cups. Add a scoop of mascarpone or clotted cream and decorate with a sprig of fresh mint.

Choose perfect cherries, strawberries or seedless grapes and dip them in melted white chocolate. When that's set, dip them again in dark bitter chocolate and chill.

Take them to bed with you and feed them to each other.

178 fruity passion

Tropical fruit has it all: redolent of steamy jungle climates (even if it actually grew in a glasshouse), it tastes, smells, looks and feels sexy. What you do with it is limited only by your imagination.

We can buy exotic fruits every day of the year. Though this has robbed them of their rarity value, the allure of forbidden fruit still clings to them. When you pull open a fig its glowing red interior and soft, juicy flesh can't help but remind you, as it did D.H. Lawrence, of "The wonderful moist conductivity towards the centre" of a woman. Ripe papayas and guavas also conceal seed-filled, scented interiors of luminous colour. Mangoes should be eaten only in the bath. It's impossible to sink your teeth into the flesh of a mango without the juice running down your chin and arms, so it seems only sensible to take off all your clothes first.

Mix an exotic fruit cocktail with clementines, fresh figs, orange sorbet (sherbet), and spiced port, as an ideal midnight snack, or a light finish to a rich meal. Just pile the fruit and sorbet into glasses, warm the port with brown sugar, cinnamon and honey, until the sugar and honey have melted, and then pour it on the fruit.

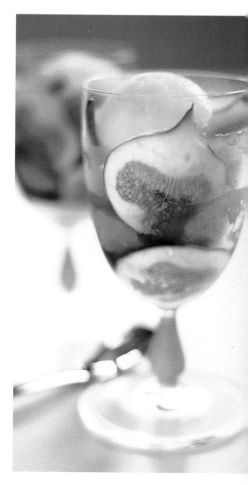

▸ *An exotic sundae can be made with any mixture of delicious fruits.*

179 popping corks

A little alcohol lowers inhibitions and increases confidence. Tease your senses with iced champagne or a voluptuous cocktail. But beware the dangers of drinking too much.

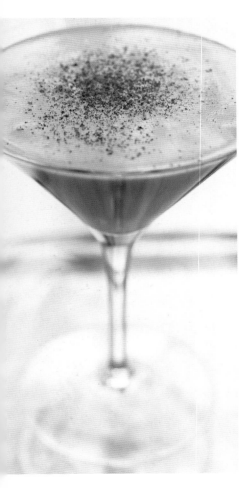

A couple of glasses of wine definitely help to create the right mood for an enjoyable romp, and could give you or your partner the confidence to try something daring and new.

Drinking wine is relaxing but it also stimulates all the senses, as you smell its complex aroma and savour its taste. As for champagne, who wouldn't feel sexier when its gentle little bubbles are tickling the nose? It envelops you in a warm, rosy glow and adds a note of celebration to the encounter – which is always flattering and romantic.

Casanova cocktail

1 measure/1 ½ tbsp bourbon
½ measure/2 tsp marsala dolce
½ measure/2 tsp Kahlua
1 measure/1 ½ tbsp double (heavy) cream

Shake all the ingredients well with plenty of ice to amalgamate the cream. Strain into a glass. Sprinkle with ground nutmeg.

◄ *This creamy cocktail looks almost as good as it tastes.*

180 aromatherapy bath oils

Turn your bathroom into a sensual haven with a gorgeously indulgent scented bath. Essential oils will get you in the mood for passion, and their scent will linger enticingly on your skin.

Just sprinkle 4-6 drops of your favourite essential oil on the surface of the water after you have drawn the bath and agitate the water to mix it. Don't add essential oils while the water is running, because much of the fragrant vapour will have dispersed before you get into the bath. If you want to soothe and moisturize dry skin, you can mix the essential oils with a carrier oil such as sweet almond, and add some wheatgerm oil which is high in skin-nourishing vitamin E.

rose and sandalwood bath oil

A little rose essential oil goes a long way, as it has a powerful fragrance. When combined with sandalwood it creates a warm, spicy fragrance.

100ml/3 ½ fl oz almond oil
20ml/4 tsp wheatgerm oil
15 drops rose essential oil
10 drops sandalwood essential oil

Pour the almond and wheatgerm oils into a bottle, add the essential oils and shake. Add a tablespoon to the bath.

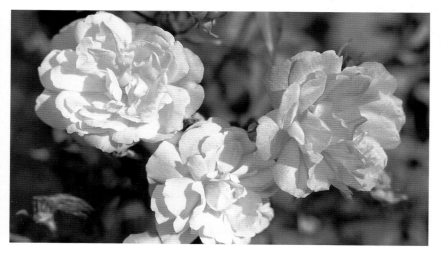

181 smooth silky skin

Toning scrubs for the face and body are great for gently exfoliating and stimulating the blood supply to the skin. They'll leave you tingling and revitalized.

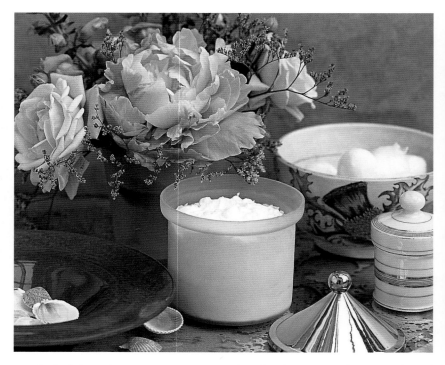

gentle facial scrub
Makes enough for 10 treatments
30ml/2 tbsp dried rose petals
45ml/3 tbsp ground almonds
45ml/3 tbsp medium oatmeal
45ml/3 tbsp powdered milk
almond oil

Powder the rose petals in a pestle and mortar or an electric grinder. Mix all the dry ingredients and store in a sealed jar. Mix to a paste with almond oil. Rub into the face, avoiding the eyes, and rinse off with warm water.

Prolong the intimacy of touch by sharing a long, indulgent bath filled with fragrant bubbles, and revel in the silky warmth caressing your skin.

183 delicious dusting powder

Don't think of talcum powder as the province of babies and old ladies. A light dusting over clean warm skin makes it feel satiny and is a wonderful way to coat the body with gentle fragrance.

You can make your own dusting powder from scratch, or use unscented talc as a base. Either way, you'll create a luxurious scented powder that's a world away from commercial brands. Pat it all over with a huge swansdown puff to make yourself feel like a star.

luscious lavender body powder
60ml/4 tbsp white kaolin clay
60ml/4 tbsp arrowroot
75ml/5 tbsp cornflour (cornstarch)
3 drops each lavender, coriander,
   lemon and geranium essential oils

Mix the kaolin, arrowroot and 60ml/4 tbsp of the cornflour. Add the essential oils to the remaining cornflour and stir into the powder.

single fragrance dusting powder
This is simple to make with ready-made unscented talc. To every 5 tablespoons of talc add 1 tablespoon of cornflour, scented with 5 drops of essential oil. Try jasmine or ylang ylang for a heavy, seductive scent, or rose for a more romantic effect.

▼ Apply your talc with a luxurious powder puff to give an extra glamorous feel.

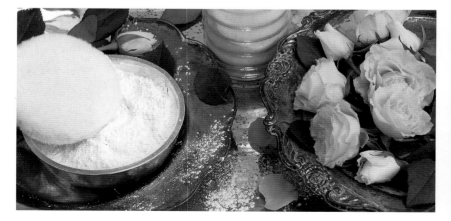

shimmering tresses

Historically, no part of a woman's body has aroused more adulation than her hair. Throughout the ages, flowing locks have been praised in poetry and celebrated in art.

The fifth-century Sanskrit poet Bhartrhari described a woman's hair as a forest, enticing the explorer into unknown territory where love waits like a bandit to ambush him. Luxuriant hair exerts a powerful sexual allure. In some cultures, it is still kept hidden to avoid tempting men.

Apart from hairdressers and masseurs, few people actually touch our heads, so running the fingers through a lover's hair is an intimate gesture. The scent of hair is personal and potent – perfume lingers longer in the hair than anywhere else, so a spritz of fragrance makes it irresistible.

Rinses made from herbs rather than chemicals give a much fresher, natural scent and will also nourish the hair.

herbal hair rinse

A simple herbal rinse gives your hair a wonderful fresh fragrance and leaves it smooth and lustrous. Pour a cup of boiling water over a handful of fresh lemon verbena leaves, or fresh parsley, and leave to infuse for at least an hour. Strain the liquid, discarding the leaves, and use as a final rinse after washing.

▾ *Herbs such as lemon verbena and parsley condition as well as scent your hair.*

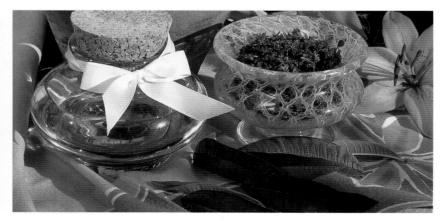

185 mint foot treatments

A foot massage can be a great turn-on. Feet are among the most sensitive areas of the body, and once you start to pamper them you may begin to see them as a seriously sexy zone.

Feet are too often tired, sore and rather neglected, but making them feel good can revitalize your whole body. Mint is a refreshing cooler for hot, aching feet and leaves them smelling sweet and feeling soothed.

mint footbath
12 large sprigs mint
120ml/4fl oz/½ cup cold water
2.4 litres/4 pints/10 cups hot water

Place the mint in a food processor with the cold water and blend to a green purée. Add to the boiling water in a large bowl and leave to cool to a bearable temperature before soaking the feet.

mint massage oil
15ml/1 tbsp almond oil
1 drop mint essential oil

Mix the oils and rub well into the feet, then begin the massage.

▼ *A massage may begin as a therapeutic exercise but lead to other things.*

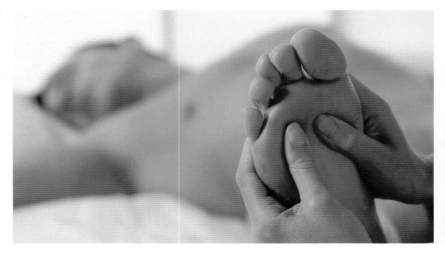

186 colour magic

People have a powerful response to colour. If you want your bedroom to feel vibrant, stimulating and just a little bit dangerous, add some cushions or throws in vibrant red.

It's impossible to be indifferent to colour. It surrounds us all the time. Its influence on mood is obvious: just imagine walking between concrete walls, sitting in the shade of a leafy tree, gazing into a clear blue sky, or putting on a bright red sweater, and you can immediately appreciate the power of colour.

feeling red

Red is the nearest visible light to heat in the electromagnetic spectrum. We connect it with heat and the danger of burning. It's the colour of smouldering coals, and lava erupting from a volcano. As the colour of blood red has links with life and liveliness. It signifies activity, daring and passion.

Phrases like "red light district" and "scarlet woman" bring out the sexual nature of red – not just sexy, but illicit – naughty rather than nice. It's an immediate colour, restless and impatient. It's associated with the expression of emotions – whether passion, anger or aggression – that can be hard to handle and make the heart beat faster, the capillaries dilate and the skin flushed and warm.

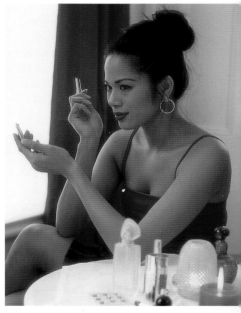

▲ Red signifies an element of danger to others, and gives you a feeling of daring.

So a red bedroom might not give you peaceful sleep, but if you want to generate vitality, boldness and passion, it's the colour to choose. Rather than painting the room red though, you could always use moveable items such as drapes and cushions.

setting the scene

Your bedroom is one of the most important rooms in your home: make it a warm cocoon of comfort and an intimate space for lovemaking and sensuality.

We spend more time in the bedroom than in any other single room, so creating the right atmosphere here can have a profound effect on how we feel all the time. The room needs to be a sanctuary, where intimate exchanges can take place in a relaxed and harmonious way.

Anything connected with the outside world should be kept to a minimum and should be out of sight. That means clearing clutter. Put clothes and shoes away, and never allow anything to do with work to creep into the bedroom. A computer is definitely a bad idea, and apart from essential items, it's better if all electrical appliances are kept somewhere else.

softness and warmth

The bed – the larger the better – clearly needs to take centre stage, without too many other pieces of furniture competing for attention. Hang billowing silk drapes or netting around the bed for a romantic, theatrical effect. A rich, sensuous haven will set the scene for intimacy, with soft, luxurious textures complemented by warm low-level lighting. Deep, warm pinks and reds are perfect, but don't use colours that are so strong and bright that you can't eventually fall into restful sleep.

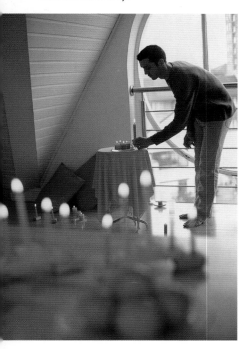

◀ *Set the scene for a night of love throughout the house, not just the bedroom.*

Make your bed a **dream** of comfort, with a **cloud-soft** duvet, the **smoothest**, coolest sheets and a mountain of **pillows**.

189 romantic lighting

The right lighting can create a magical space, whether you're preparing the bathroom for an evening of sensual solitude or setting the scene for seduction in the bedroom.

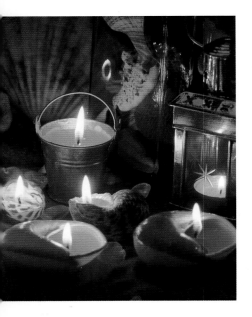

◀ *Candlelight can't be beaten for creating a beautiful glow, and a relaxing atmosphere.*

Fairylights or christmas lights also cast a gentle but exciting light and are very flattering. String them around the bedhead to lend enchantment and magic to the proceedings.

seashell candles
You can scent these enchanting little candles by adding a seductive essential oil to the wax.
clean shells
sand–filled bowl
150g/5oz paraffin wax
50g/2oz natural beeswax
double boiler
metal–core wick for small candles
waxed paper

The warm glow of candlelight is the most flattering of all, smoothing away imperfections and giving skin a luminous sheen. Flickering candle flames have a hypnotic, relaxing effect. Create an extravagant, fantastic scene by filling the room with candles, or light just a few near the bed for an intimate, cavelike effect in an otherwise darkened room.

1 Steady the shells in the sand-filled bowl. Melt the waxes together in a double boiler. Prime the wicks by soaking the lengths in the wax and leave to cool on waxed paper.

2 Pour the hot wax into the shells (do not overfill). Leave until partially set then push in the primed wicks.

190 scents for seduction

The sense of smell is the most primitive of our five senses, and perfumes of all kinds are powerful triggers of both physical and emotional responses. Scent and sex are inextricably linked.

Legend has it that Mark Antony had to wade through a carpet of rose petals in order to reach Cleopatra's bed, and perfume is a traditional gift of love. But the scent most strongly redolent of sex is the natural smell of bodies.

erogenic scents

Like plants and animals, a natural aroma is part of our biological strategy for attracting a mate. Hormone-like chemicals, known as pheromones, are scent signals radiated by the skin. Certain animal and plant fragrances resemble human pheromones, and can be used to stimulate sexual desire. They are known as erogenic aromas.

Musk, a secretion of the musk deer, is probably the most famous, with its earthy, sensuous scent. Erogenic aromas are also found in jasmine, rose, ylang ylang and patchouli.

using scent

The bedroom can be subtly scented with fragrant oils, scented candles or flowers. Scatter rose petals on the bed, scent linen when you wash and iron it, and spray perfume in a fine mist over the carpet so that the fragrance is released when you walk on it.

▼ Scent your bedroom with fresh flower heads and bowls of essential oils.

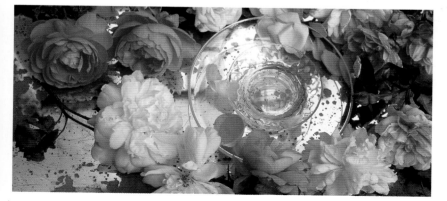

191 sexy essential oils

Essential oils can be used in many ways to cast their spell on your senses. They are concentrated substances, each with its own characteristics and properties, and their effects can be profound.

The erotic charge of these aromas has made them famous as ingredients of love potions and perfume blends designed for seduction. Use them in aromatherapy burners, in oil blends for massage or to fragrance baths.

jasmine
The warm, exotic smell of jasmine has a musky undertone, and has been used for centuries in love potions and bridal garlands. Its euphoric effect can liberate sexual fantasies.

ylang ylang
The relaxing effect of this intensely sweet scent reduces stress levels and removes inhibition.

neroli
Orange blossom is reputed to raise the libido, lull inhibitions and allow secret desires to be expressed.

clary sage
This heady, sweet aroma has a euphoric and relaxing effect.

▸ *Establish an aromatherapy burner in your room and a selection of essential oils.*

sandalwood
Probably the oldest perfume in history, sandalwood's heavy scent can lift depression that often causes sexual problems.

rose
The rose is a symbol of love and romantic longing. Its wonderful fragrance evokes general feelings of pleasure and happiness.

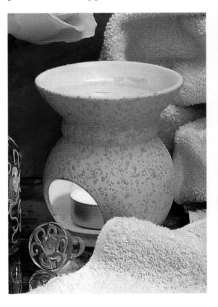

192 pillow talk

Talking about your innermost feelings can be difficult, but one of the most successful ways to keep a relationship flourishing is by being best friends and being open with each other.

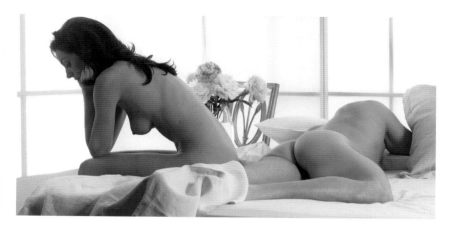

It takes time to build up trust and feel able to talk about your fantasies, fears and needs, but communication is key in every relationship. It's important to let the other person know what you are feeling or expecting, not just to avoid misunderstandings but to get what you want.

Are there things you'd love your partner to try? Is there something a little perverse that you'd like to do during sex but are too embarrassed to suggest? Is there anything you don't really like your partner doing, but don't want to mention?

▲ Communication is vital for a healthy relationship and an active sex life.

sexual communication

Direct criticism can be upsetting and intimidating. The best way to tell your partner about your likes and dislikes is by affirmation: "I love it when you touch me there," for example, or "It feels better this way." Once you've opened a channel of communication in this positive way, it may be easier to talk about things that are a problem for you, and to open the way for your partner to do the same.

193 loving face massage

Slowly, gently massaging your lover's face with awareness and sensitivity can be a very intimate, sensual experience for both of you. Enhance the massage by using some essential oils.

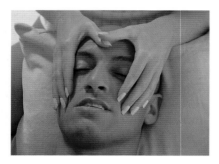

1 Apply a small quantity of oil to your hands. Use them to stroke gently, one after the other, first up over the neck, and then across the chin and jaw, up to the forehead. Glide your thumbs steadily from the centre of the brow towards the sides of the head. Repeat the stroke up over the entire forehead. Rotate your fingertips anti-clockwise on one place all over the cheeks.

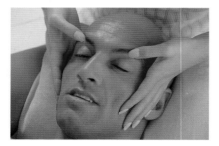

2 Draw your thumbs from the inner to the outer edges of the eyebrows, then press the pads sensitively up into and along the brow bone. Repeat the movement down the nose, beginning at the bridge and moving your thumbs down to the nostrils then out towards the cheekbones.

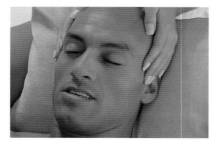

3 Relax your hands to sweep the palms soothingly up over the sides of the temples and scalp, then draw them away from the head. Softly cup your hands, circling your fingertips several times in soothing clockwise motions over your partner's temples. Complete the massage by cradling the head between your hands.

194 sensual touch

The most important element of sensual massage is the caring presence of your hands on your partner's body. Allow your intuition to show you how and where to apply the strokes.

After a stressful day, massaging your partner allows you time to wind down and get back in touch with one another. It need not be a precursor to sex, but it can set the scene and get you both in the mood.

Pour a little oil into your hands and warm them by rubbing them together before you begin. Long, sweeping strokes over the back can be performed while straddling your partner's hips. This keeps you in close contact, but you should support your own weight. Maintain a constant, confident touch, using long, flowing unbroken strokes. Your hands should encompass fully the contours of the body, such as the shoulders, hips and buttocks.

▾ Your touch can be at times soft, gentle and nurturing or firm and stimulating.

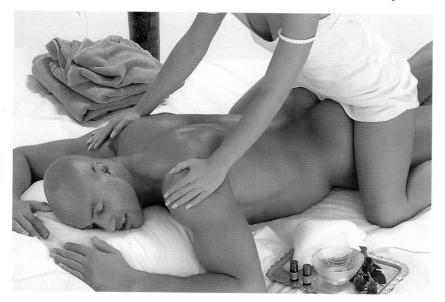

195 kissing asides

There's a whole repertoire of kissing to try out: not all kisses have to involve tickling each other's tonsils. In the right circumstances an almost imperceptible brush of the lips can be just as exciting.

Women tend to like kissing better than men, and enjoy the whole, long, lingering embrace, without it necessarily leading on to anything else. Some women say that they find kissing the most erotic part of sex, whereas men tend to see it as a step on the way to intercourse. What makes a great kiss? Here are a few suggestions:

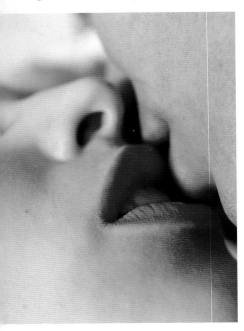

french kissing: Gently caress the inside of your partner's mouth with your tongue. As they respond, you can quicken the pace and intensity, going for a fuller thrust.

chicken kisses: Great for moments of tenderness. Plant light pecks at the rate of about three a second. It's between a kiss and a tickle, but feels good.

stereophonic kiss: Some people adore the sound and sensation of being kissed inside their ears – the slooshing sound really turns them on.

talking kiss: Hold your partner's face between your hands and kiss different parts of it – each eyebrow, each eyelid, nose, cheeks – and between each kiss say something erotic: what you're about to do to them, what you'd like them to do to you, and so on.

butterfly kiss: Use your eyelashes to brush against your partner's face or body.

love bites: Think twice before you bite, they hurt.

◀ *Kissing sometimes gets abandoned in a long established relationship. Try and revive it if that is the case in yours.*

Play with an ice cube: try sliding it over your bodies, passing it from mouth to mouth. The sensation of iced water against hot skin excites nerve endings in a way that hands and fingers can't.

For a truly sensual experience, take a journey around your partner's body. Think of it as a luscious and varied landscape: instead of the familiar places, visit the parts you've hardly explored.

How often has your partner absently stroked the inside of your wrist, sending electrifying spasms through your body? Sometimes the less obvious parts of the body create the biggest thrills. Focusing on different areas shows that you find your partner sexy all over, not just at the hotspots.

erogenous zones

The back of the neck is a very relaxing and loving place to caress a lover, as it has a mysterious link to the body's sensual centres. It sends a mixture of warm and thrilling shock waves along the entire length of the spine, leaving you feeling energized and loved.

The navel is another extremely sensitive area. Some people are a bit squeamish about it, but others love having their belly buttons caressed by a soft tongue.

Fingers are an understandably popular focus of attention, because their tips are so sensitive, and sucking the fingers is loaded with innuendo. The toes are just as sensitive, but sucking them is something that people either love or hate. Some find it a real turn-on. For those who can

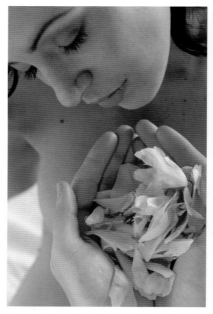

▲ Taking time to explore each others' bodies will help your love-making.

bear to have their feet touched, the instep is another nerve-rich area. Many people love to have their feet massaged and pampered. Using your toes can also be an interesting way to stimulate other areas of your partner's body (as long as your feet aren't cold).

198 playing games

Sex isn't something that needs to be taken seriously, it should be fun. If things are becoming repetitive in your relationship, it's time to spice up your love-making with some fun and games.

There are lots of possibilities: you can play strip poker, naked Scrabble, or hide and seek. Why not adapt the rules of the games and introduce some forfeits of your own?

dice game

Get two dice. Write down a sexual position for each number on the first die. Then write down six locations for the second. Roll the dice together and obey dutifully.

▼ *Ring your partner on his mobile from the bedroom and indulge in some sex talk.*

sex with a stranger

Here's an idea for an anniversary surprise. Invite your partner to meet you for a meal, both pretending you are strangers on a blind date.

Spend the evening flirting as you did when you first met. At the end of the evening suggest a one-night stand in the hotel room nearby (that you've already secretly booked). If you can stay in character, playing the consummate sexual host or hostess and doing anything your partner requests, this should guarantee some passionate and exciting sex.

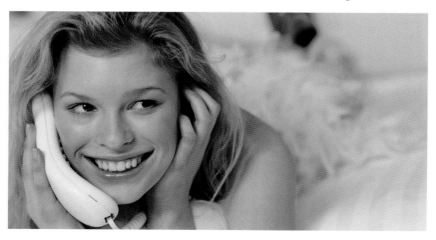

199 erotica

Reading erotic literature stimulates the erogenous zone that full-on pornography simply can't reach – the brain. Read it alone, or together, or to each other, for a great turn-on.

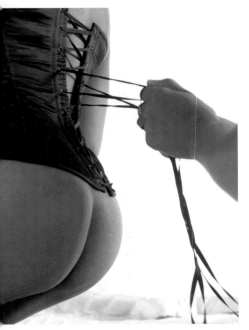

▲ The simplest prop can instantly conjure up a storm of sexual meaning.

Erotic literature and films can be a great aid to sex, whether you use them as a warm-up act beforehand or read them together in bed. The choice of novels, poetry and magazines is huge these days. They can provide you with ready-made scenarios to act out between you, or inspire and embellish your own fantasies.

Your favourite sensual or erotic films are guaranteed to get you in the mood: you might be inspired by a raunchy modern sex scene or by the buttoned-up restraint of a costume drama, where desire has to smoulder under the surface.

pornography

At the other end of the scale, gritty porn films and dirty magazines can be exciting because of their complete lack of subtlety. They can help you express desires and fantasies that you would probably never act upon. They might even give you some interesting ideas, or they might just make you roar with laughter together.

If you have a camcorder you could try making your own porn film. Choose your roles and dress up appropriately, position the camera with a good view of the bed and off you go. Watching it afterwards can be extremely erotic – seeing yourselves making love from a different angle gives you a whole new perspective.

200 sharing fantasies

People guard their fantasies fiercely, regardless of how close they are to their partner. It can be liberating to share some of yours with your lover, and even more so to act them out.

Humans have very complex brains, and it's often not enough just to stimulate the genitals to feel sexually fulfilled. We have to be in just the correct mood before we are relaxed enough to let our bodies go, and our personal fantasies can provide the right mind-set.

Some fantasies are simple enough to enact: having sex in an exclusive and elegant hotel, being wooed in a romantic candlelit room, or being swept away by passion on a warm and sunny cliff-top. Others that involve a cast of thousands, all acting in the way your fantasy requires, aren't so easy.

Having sex with a celebrity is a common fantasy. If you try this one while having sex with your partner it won't do any harm – as long as you don't scream out the wrong name at the wrong time.

private thoughts

Many people are embarassed by the content of their fantasies, and worry that they imagine weird or illegal acts, but it's worth remembering that it's human instinct to be drawn precisely to whatever's forbidden.

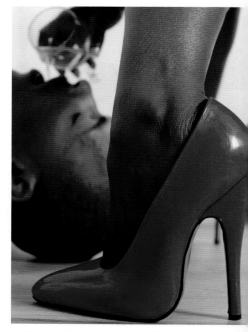

▲ A fantasy that you share might become an enjoyable part of your sex life.

Keep your fantasies as a private store of erotic movies that you can switch on whenever you like. Your brain is the biggest and most powerful sex organ you have and where the mind leads, the body will follow.

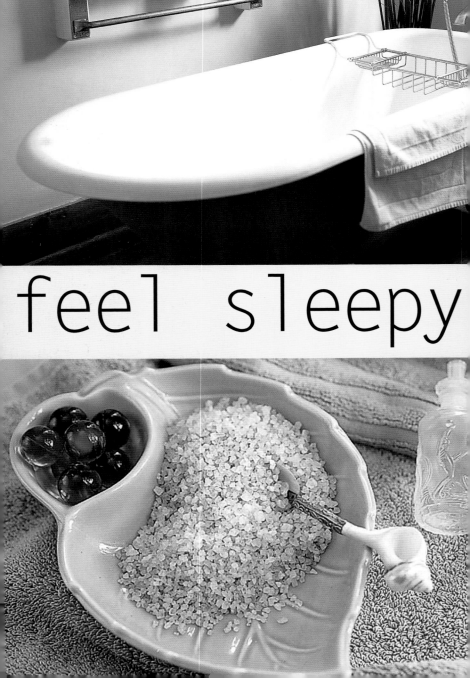

feel sleepy

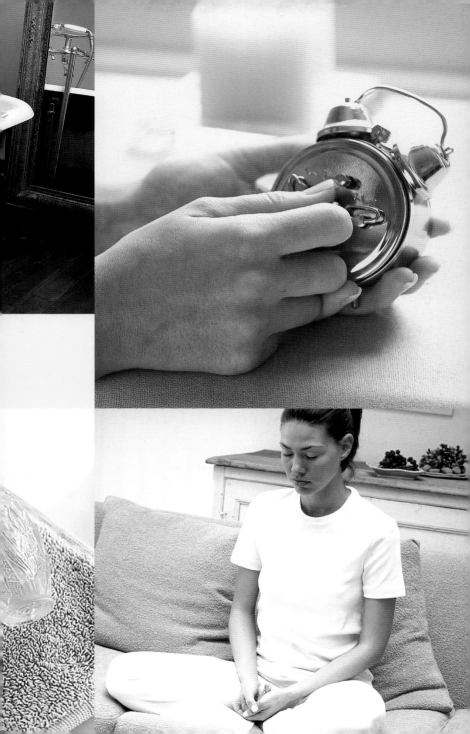

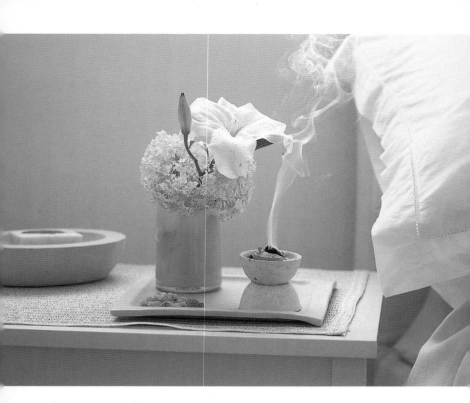

learn the secrets of better sleep

The average adult spends between seven and nine hours asleep each night. We know that during this time, the body makes any necessary repairs. Toxins are eliminated, tissues and cells are rebuilt. The mind processes stress that has accumulated during the waking hours, reducing its adverse effect on the system. But even with extensive research in the laboratory, many of the functions of sleep remain a mystery. One thing is certain, though – without it, the body and mind cannot operate properly. If sleep is missed or of poor quality for long periods of time, both our physical and mental health suffer. Sleep deprivation takes its toll on your productivity, your enjoyment of life and your looks.

Fortunately, there are many effective ways to stave off temporary bouts of insomnia and ensure continual deep sleep, night after night, allowing you to work and play at optimum energy levels.

exercise to relax

Keeping the body moving is essential for good sleep – without exercise, you will not be physically tired enough to rest at night. Aerobic activities such as

◀ A bedroom that is calm and peaceful will help you to relax at bedtime.

walking and cycling exercise the heart and tone the muscles, while some specific yoga techniques provide an excellent way to stretch and relax.

balance and perspective

At certain times, insomnia may result from stress. Massage techniques can ease tense necks, aching shoulders and uptight torsos, and face massage can be an instant calmer.

Some stress is an inevitable part of life, but when you need to achieve a state of inner calm, a range of meditation and visualization techniques can help you work through your insecurities, worries and anxieties. With practice, stress can be diminished so that it is no longer a cause of sleepless nights.

a calm environment

Lack of sleep can also be exacerbated by external factors such as noise, a "busy" atmosphere in the bedroom, or simply the wrong type of mattress. By making the best of your physical environment, you can reduce or remove many of these detrimental factors.

Following the principles of feng shui you can arrange your bedroom space to best effect and remove clutter that can clog free-flowing "chi" or energy. Choosing a calming room decor and lighting scheme can soothe the senses, while establishing a bedtime ritual can make sleep a pleasant and comforting experience to look forward to.

pampering treatments

In view of the many demands made by daily life, it is essential to find time to switch off from cares and worries in the evening, and indulge in some personal quality time. However busy you are, you should take time to wind down before trying to go to sleep, otherwise your mind will still be buzzing with the concerns of the day. Surrounding yourself with gentle

▼ A massage from your partner will help to ensure a good night's sleep.

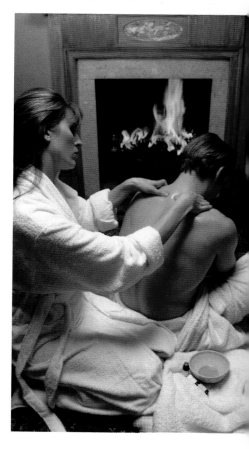

candlelight and sinking into a hot bath laced with aromatherapy oils or herbal sachets can go a long way to soothe and prepare your body for sleep. Essential oils such as lavender and clary sage added to the water help to diminish tension headaches and muscular aches, while bath bags or bath salts made with chamomile help to ease stress. You can also use the natural energies from flowers and herbs as a base for warming foot baths, soporific sleep pillows and effective sleep tinctures.

bedtime snacks

You ate dinner at 6pm; it's now 11:30pm and you're ready to go to bed, but now you're feeling hungry and thirsty again. What do you do? Instead of raiding the refrigerator for a substantial and perhaps indigestible

▾ A cup of fragrant chamomile tea at bedtime will help you drift off to sleep.

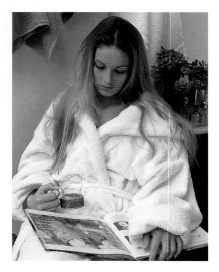

meal, it is better to opt for a light snack, such as toast with a topping, and perhaps a hot, comforting beverage. Try to avoid tea and coffee as they are stimulants and will tend to keep you awake if you drink them late in the day. Instead, herbal teas prepared for their sedative properties may be sipped in the evening, while warm, milky drinks are ideal for consumption before bed – milk contains peptides that calm the system. The occasional hot toddy can also provide a delicious way to wind down, and this is particularly good on a cold winter's evening, especially if you are suffering from a cold.

calming the psyche

Sometimes it is difficult to sleep due to excessive emotions, such as fear, excitement or anxiety. Crystal therapy can help to calm heartache; choosing the right stones can also calm restlessness and anxiety, and help to regulate sleep patterns. Crystals can be helpful when bad dreams and nightmares are keeping you awake, as can techniques such as visualizing a guardian angel or spiritual protector. When you have perplexing or mysti-fying dreams, it can be very helpful to write down what happened before you forget, so that you can ponder and try to analyse them later on. Working towards an understanding of your dreams adds an enjoyable richness to what can be the fascinating pageant of sleep.

▸ Make bathtime special with soft candlelight and fragrant oils.

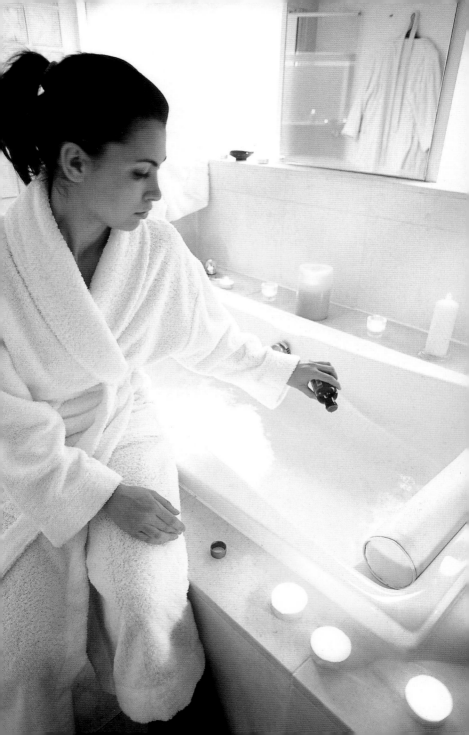

sleep treatments

This chapter is divided into sections that address different ways to achieve healthy sleep using natural remedies and techniques. It is designed so that you can select from many options to aid a state of rest, from relaxation techniques and aromatherapy baths, to creating the right bedroom atmosphere, to meditation and dream work.

To keep your body supple and relaxed, massage, reflexology and yoga techniques are suggested. A section on aromatherapy explores ways to relieve tension and irritation, and to rid the system of damaging anger and stress, while recipes for bath salts, sleep pillows and herbal teas are designed to soothe you to sleep.

Finally, esoteric sleep aids and quick fixes – from healing and calming crystals, to techniques for exploring and understanding your dreams – help to bring calm and balance to your sleeping and waking life. And if all else fails, try instant cures, such as sniffing an onion – which just might work.

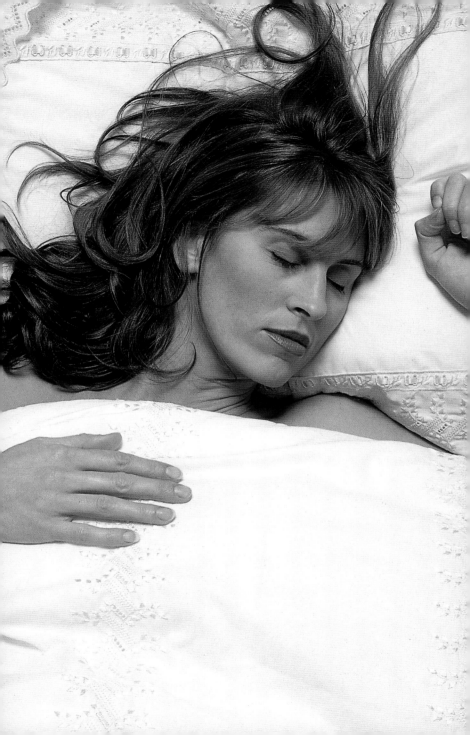

201 releasing emotional stress

Stress from daily life can affect us negatively, while the effects of an accident or shock can last a long time. One of the most effective ways to release stress is through the frontal eminences of the skull.

1 Lightly hold your fingertips to the frontal eminences of your skull, the two slight bumps above the outer edge of the eye at either side of your forehead. Alternatively, hold a hand across your forehead to catch both points easily.

2 Turning your attention to the stressful event will now automatically begin to release the accumulated tensions. It is not necessary to relive each aspect of the event in detail,

though often this occurs automatically. Strong feelings and emotions, as well as physical reaction, may surface while these points are being held, so expect to feel emotional.

3 As long as the process is allowed to complete itself, the body quickly and effectively releases the frozen memories once and for all.

▼ *The effects of shock can last beyond the actual event, colouring our lives for years.*

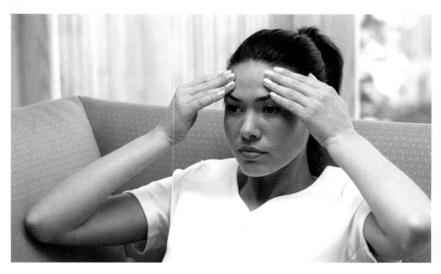

202 tense neck easer

When you are fatigued, aching, tense muscles in the neck and shoulders make it difficult to get comfortable in bed. Use these self-massage techniques to target problem areas for fast relief.

1 Start by shrugging your shoulders then letting them relax completely a few times. Firmly grip your opposite shoulder with your hand and use a squeezing motion to loosen tension. Repeat on the other shoulder. This kneading action removes waste matter from tired muscles and moves fresh, oxygenated blood into them.

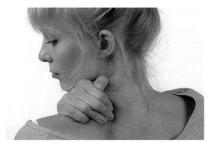

2 With the fingers of both hands, grip the back of the neck and squeeze in a circular motion to relax the muscles leading up either side of the neck. Work up to the base of the skull and down again to the shoulders.

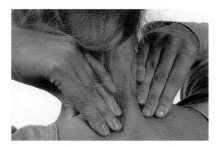

3 Move the thumbs in a circular movement across the neck and right up to the base of the skull. You should feel the bone as you apply moderate pressure. Rest for a few moments before standing and moving.

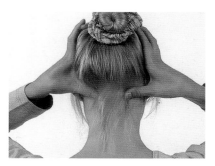

203 daily exercise

Some kind of physical exercise during the day is essential for a good night's sleep. Humans are designed to move – it is no use expecting to sleep easily and deeply if your body isn't tired.

Making time for exercise is of the utmost importance for a healthy lifestyle. Many people in sedentary occupations feel that they have no time for exercise, or are too tired at the end of the day. Exercise not only boosts physical stamina, but it also enhances your mental outlook and self esteem, through the release of endorphins, hormones that foster a positive mood. It also builds muscle tissue, and as you grow in physical strength, you will also feel stronger mentally and emotionally.

Spend as much time as possible outdoors, as sunlight helps to regulate the body clock. This is especially important during the short days of winter, when natural light will help to keep depression and SAD (Seasonal Affective Disorder) at bay.

Walking can be done almost anywhere, and it helps to keep the heart and other organs healthy. Activities such as swimming, tennis, squash, weight-lifting and dancing require more thought and planning, but they offer tremendous rewards and are very enjoyable. Whichever activity you choose, aim to exercise for at least 45 minutes three times a week – but for optimum fitness and to ensure restful sleep, try to make time for some exercise every day.

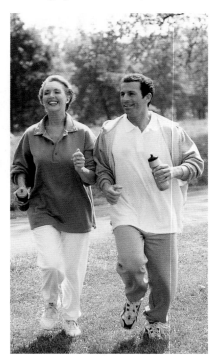

◀ *Jogging gets you out in the sun and fresh air, as well as exercising the lungs and heart.*

To relieve tension and enhance restfulness before retiring to bed, massage the web between your thumb and index finger on both hands.

205 yoga stressbuster

Used to calm the body and channel the mind, yoga is an excellent way to de-stress. The following technique focuses the mind on relaxing every part of the body.

Lie on your back with a bolster of blankets arranged under your upper body so that your shoulders are slightly elevated; this "opens" your upper chest and your lungs to allow free breathing (this is called the Savasana position). Spend a few minutes relaxing the body. Release tension from the feet and hands, the abdomen and face.

Calm your thoughts as you focus your mind on each part of your upper body in turn. Keep the eyes still and let the eyeballs relax down into the eye sockets. Relax the temples and forehead. Relax the bridge of the nose. Relax the cheeks by releasing them away from the eyes, then the jaws, moving the lower jaw a little way from the upper without tensing it.

Feel the connection between the ear passages and the jaws, and relax them. Keep the tongue still, letting it rest on the lower palate; allow the root of the tongue to recede into the throat, keeping the teeth lightly parted.

Next, relax your neck and throat by pressing the shoulders down and moving the shoulder blades into the back ribs. At the same time, bring the chin slightly down towards the throat. Quiet the vibrations of your vocal cords. End your relaxation here. Before getting up, turn on to your right side, with knees close to the chest and remain resting there for a moment or two.

▾ *Follow a simple yoga relaxation routine to unwind completely after a busy day.*

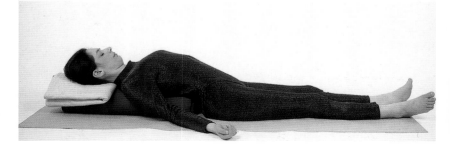

206 sensual massage

By learning basic massage strokes, you and your partner can touch each other with tenderness, sensuality and playfulness, relaxing each other's body and mind, enhancing the ability to sleep.

1 Begin by making sure the place you are going to massage your partner is warm and comfortable. With your partner lying on their front, sit at the top of their body. Put some oil in your hands, then place them on either side of the spine, and glide down the back. Move out to the sides and up the back again; repeat several times.

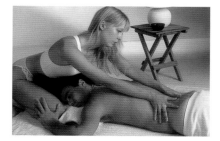

2 With a gentle motion, stroke down the centre of the back, with one hand following the other smoothly, as if you were stroking a cat. As one hand lifts off the small of the back, start again with the other at the neck. Continue this movement for several minutes.

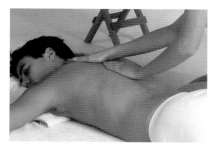

3 Place both hands on the upper back and stroke outwards in a fan shape. Work down the back and buttocks, using the fanning action.

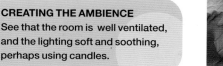

CREATING THE AMBIENCE
See that the room is well ventilated, and the lighting soft and soothing, perhaps using candles.

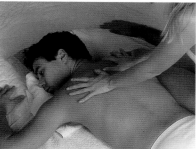

207 body & mind balancing

Learning to relax is crucial for maintaining a healthy body and mind. By letting go of tension, you will achieve a state of balance that allows easy and satisfying sleep, night after night.

Along with a nutritious diet, an exercise programme and a positive attitude, relaxation will help you keep your balance and perspective, even at those times when being under pressure is unavoidable. It can be beneficial to do the following exercise in the early evening, when you come home from your job or have finished your chores for the day. You can also use this technique to give yourself a midday oasis of serenity, if you can find a quiet place to stretch out for ten minutes. Deep, steady breathing will oxygenate your bloodstream, relieving stress on all the organs, including the brain, thus helping the thinking processes.

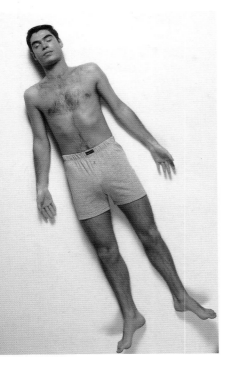

whole body relaxation
Lie down in a straight line, with shoulders relaxed and aligned on the floor. The arms should be straight – but not rigid – with elbows alongside the waist, palms turned upwards. Relax your head and close your eyes. Breathe in deeply down to your diaphragm (lower abdomen), and allow your body to sink into the floor. Breathe out slowly and relax. Focus attention on your breathing: listen as you inhale and exhale, and notice how quiet your deep breathing can become.

◀ *A daily ten-minute period of relaxation relieves stress and helps clear the mind.*

208 meditative visualization

Meditating can help bring mind and body into a state of harmony. It is a way to balance an active life with calming periods of inner reflection, and has the benefit of promoting easy, restful sleep.

Regular meditation, combined with positive affirmations, can help you to "centre" your mind, alleviating stress and allowing you to see a clear way forward through the daily problems and challenges you may face.

ease into meditation

Choose a quiet place for meditating, one where you won't be interrupted. Get into a comfortable position: sitting cross-legged is a traditional pose, but you may sit in a comfortable chair. Close your eyes, breathe deeply with your hands resting on your lap, and allow all thoughts to slowly leave your mind, as sand trickles through the neck of an hourglass. You may wish to focus on a word, or mantra, such as "OM": repeat this over and over until tension has left your body and mind. Or you could visualize a colour, allowing it to surround and suffuse you with its calming rays.

Allow 10 to 20 minutes each time you meditate; doing this twice daily is an effective way to restore composure. Informal meditation can be done any time you need a break; close your eyes for a few minutes and breathe deeply.

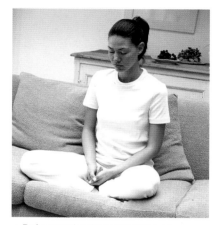

▲ *Before you begin meditating, make sure that you are relaxed and comfortable.*

AFFIRMATIONS

Speak or read these affirmations each night when you go to bed to remind yourself of your inner strengths before going to sleep.

• I enjoyed solving the problems I dealt with today, having done the best I could do.

• I enjoyed being calm and patient today, even when others were not.

• I will sleep deeply and peacefully, to awake in the morning fresh and full of energy.

209 leaving troubles behind

This meditation is sometimes called the "railway tunnel". Designed to help you focus on the present and leave you unfettered by past worries, it can be a very effective means of paving the way to sleep.

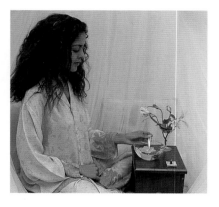

◀ It helps to clear your mind of all thoughts before you begin the meditation.

Imagine strolling along a path between two high banks, with a dull, cloudy sky above … a heavy back-pack makes your steps heavy and slow. … You trudge along, feeling damp and cold. You reach the entrance to an old railway tunnel … It is very dark, but you can see a point of light at the end, which is reassuring.… As you enter, all your self-doubts begin to surface … you are aware of your failings and regrets.… Let them rise gently to the surface of your mind. The back-pack is getting lighter as they surface.

There is a pool of light on the floor ahead from an air shaft. As you go through the light, you remember a happy time, when you felt really good about yourself. As you move into the darkness again, you feel lighter; your back-pack is emptying, but the doubts are rising to the surface once more.… The circle of light at the end of the tunnel is growing, but here is another air shaft. As you pass through the light, another good memory comes into your mind. Now you are back in the gloom, but it doesn't seem as intense as before. It is getting lighter and warmer, and you experience more good memories.… As you near the end, you notice that the sun has come out, and you feel as if your load has disappeared. Warmth begins to replace the cold you felt before.

Eventually, you step out into the sunshine with a light tread, valuing yourself and the world much more. You realize you have so many opportunities awaiting you, and new chances to accomplish things. Your contribution is important, and you are a valuable and lovable person.

210 steps to sleep

The following visualization is similar to the traditional sleep cure of "counting sheep". Try taking a few deep breaths before beginning, as you prepare to let go of the day's cares.

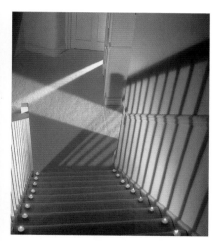

◄ Visualize a staircase, inviting you down into a state of complete relaxation.

stairway visualization

Imagine taking the first steps down, relaxing and letting go, feeling beautifully at ease and at peace. On step 8, you are becoming more relaxed ... on step 7, you are drifting deeper ... and deeper ... down still.

By step 6, you are calmer ... and calmer.... Halfway down, you are letting go and feeling good. On step 4, you are relaxing even more ... By step 3, you are sinking deeper.

On step 2, you are enjoying pleasant, peaceful feelings, half-awake, half-asleep. On step 1, you are feeling beautifully relaxed. On reaching the the bottom, you are so pleasantly relaxed, you can allow your mind to drift into sleep....

Imagine a staircase stretching down in front of you, made up of ten steps covered in soft, natural-coloured carpet, perhaps lit with candles or lanterns. You are standing on the tenth step. Count backwards from 10 to 0, and as you count backwards, imagine each number as a step, and each step as a step down the staircase into deeper and deeper levels of relaxation, so that by the time you get to 0, you can allow yourself to be as deeply relaxed as you can manage, while still being aware of the sounds around you.

VISUALIZATION TIPS
• Make sure you are warm and comfortable before you begin.
• If distracting thoughts enter your mind during the visualization, just let them drift on out.

instant relaxation

Once you begin to experience the positive effects of meditation, you can utilize "triggers" – evocative words and images that take you back into a state of relaxation – during the day or to aid sleep.

If you have imagined being in a certain place, or speaking a certain word or phrase during meditation, you can do so again to evoke the same positive feelings. For example, you may have imagined yourself sitting near a peaceful lake: if you conjure up that image again during a stressful meeting or a traffic jam, the memory will help you to relax instantly.

Repeating words or catch-phrases that mean much to you – such as "field of flowers" or "entering the dream" – can have the same calming effect, and will bring an instant pause to stress. If you are lying in bed, restless, be patient and pursue the image or word until you are enveloped in a sense of calm.

trigger happy

You may be aware of certain physical symptoms during meditation, such as a tingling sensation in the hands or feet: this can be a useful trigger, too. Imagine that you feel those symptoms, and within seconds you will gain the feelings associated with meditation. This can be especially useful before an important meeting, or on any occasion

about which you may be feeling a little apprehensive.

Use the triggers to gain the calm confidence you need and to put things into their proper perspective. With practice, your mind will accept the linkages you have created, and will respond to these signals at any time, quickly and easily, giving you instant access to all the benefits that come with deep contemplation.

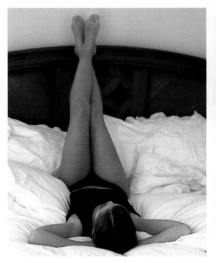

▲ Use the triggers acquired in meditation to achieve calm whenever you need it.

When future tasks are keeping you awake at night, free your mind by writing a "to do" list of things you need to accomplish tomorrow.

213 the serene bedroom

The bedroom is one of the most important rooms in the house. The Chinese principles of feng shui can help you to arrange it so that the room is suitable for relaxing, regeneration and romance.

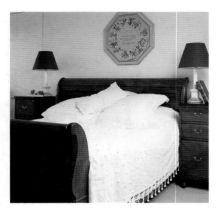

◄ Ideally, mattresses should be raised off the floor and made from natural materials.

Harmful electromagnetic waves – even from clock radios – can have an adverse effect on sleep.

Overall symmetry is important: side tables should complement each other's positions, and pictures should be hung in pairs. Photographs of parents, children and friends should have no place in a couple's private space. Mirrors in the bedroom should not face the bed. The Chinese believe that the soul leaves the body when we sleep and will become disconcerted if it comes across itself in a mirror.

We spend about a third of our lives in bed, so it is fundamental to make the bedroom peaceful and relaxed. Feng shui governs the placing of furniture and objects so that "chi", or energy, can flow in the most propitious way. It enhances a serene environment.

The best position for the bed is diagonally opposite the door, so that you can see who is entering the room. If a line of chi between the door and a window crosses the bed, it is thought to cause illness.

Keep electrical equipment out of the bedroom completely, as it detracts from the main function of the room.

CLEARING CLUTTER
Clear unnecessary clutter from the bedroom to create a sense of calm and enhance the flow of chi:
- Medicine bottles
- Cosmetics
- Used tissues
- Piles of clothes
- Old unworn clothes and shoes
- Full waste bins
- Work and papers
- TVs and music systems

a relaxing space

The physical set-up of the bedroom can go a long way towards helping you wind down at the end of the day. From lighting schemes to mattresses, you can facilitate maximum relaxation.

▸ *Use soft lighting beside your bed rather than harsh overhead lights.*

The most important item of furniture in the bedroom is the bed itself: a comfortable, supportive mattress is essential for restorative sleep. Shop around carefully for one that suits your weight and build. If a mattress is too soft or too firm, not only might it prevent peaceful slumber, it may be bad for your back as well. The surface should support your spine but give slightly. If you buy a mattress and find – after a trial week or two – that you've made a mistake, it is best to give in and buy another.

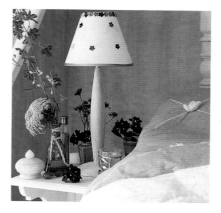

clouds of colour

Swathing your room in peaceful colours such as ivory, sky blue or delicate rose can have a wonderfully calming effect on the nervous system. Soft furnishings such as curtains and bedlinen should be soft, luxurious and tactile. Use only natural materials, they last longer than synthetics and "breathe" more easily.

Choose a lighting scheme that optimizes rest. Veto harsh, overhead lights in favour of small lamps. Try amber or soft-light bulbs of low wattage, keeping a brighter directional lamp at your bedside for reading. Candles are very soothing and can aid meditation and winding down, but remember to blow them out before you go to sleep.

RELAXATION TIPS
• Don't keep computers or work in the bedroom, as you will be unable to forget the cares of the day.
• Read a relaxing book. A tense thriller may keep you awake.

215 soothing bedtime ritual

As you approach bedtime, carrying out a familiar ritual – one on which you needn't spend much thought – is part of the process of shifting gears down towards sleep.

Many people find that a bedtime routine – such as taking a leisurely bath, preparing a hot drink and reading poetry – makes bedtime comforting and familiar. If you have children, your own rituals will be even more precious as a method of easing into slumber once you have said goodnight to them. This is your own time to enjoy peace and privacy.

Once you have decided to turn in for the night, unwelcome intrusions from other housemates or family members can be deterred by hanging

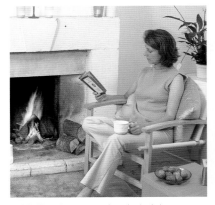
▲ Making time to read and wind down before you go to bed can be beneficial.

a "do not disturb" sign on the door. If friends often telephone late, don't bother taking the call – let the answering machine take them.

Music or your favourite late-night radio programme can ease your mind before sleep. If you like to read in bed, allow yourself time for it and go to bed earlier so you get as much sleep as you need. It can be comforting to keep favourite images or objects near your bed and glance at them before you sleep, to remind you of people you love and happy times.

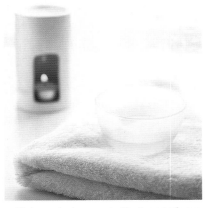
▲ Make a relaxing scented bath part of your regular evening routine.

a winding down bedtime ritual

To end the day, you can use this modified version of a ritual that has its origins in the teachings of the cabbala, an immensely powerful Hebrew magical system.

Before you begin the ritual, calm and centre yourself. Stand facing west – the direction of the setting sun – and for a few moments relate to the sun sinking down on the horizon, whether it is actually still daylight or already dark.

Imagine a beam of brilliant white light shining down on you from an infinite height. As it touches your head, it transforms your entire body into light-filled glass, like a clear bottle of human shape. As the light courses down through your body, it changes hue, moving through all the colours of the rainbow. As these colours flow down, imagine any dark areas of your body being cleansed by the rainbow light pushing the blackness down and out through the soles of your feet. As it flows out of your feet, imagine that it is forming a pool or puddle of black mire, and that this pool is then draining away into nothingness, leaving you clean and filled with brilliant, opalescent, rainbow hues.

To add to the effectiveness of the ritual and enhance your ability to sleep, place an amethyst or clear quartz crystal under your pillow before you settle down to sleep.

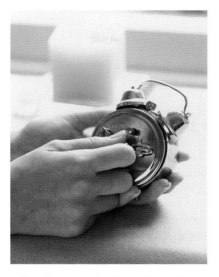

▲ If you have a set time for waking each morning your body will soon find a routine.

a dreaming tea mix

Mix the following herbs to make up a relaxing tea that can help you to have a restful night's sleep and to recall your dreams. Sip the tea about half an hour before you go to sleep. (It is not advisable to drink this tea if you are pregnant.)

1 heaped tsp jasmine flowers
1 heaped tsp chamomile flowers
2 sprigs fresh marjoram
a large cup or mug of boiled water

Place all the herbs in a jug and pour over the boiled water. Leave to infuse for 5 minutes, then strain into a cup and sweeten with honey if desired.

tuning out the noise

Noise has an increasing presence in life, whether from neighbours, machines, dogs, road traffic or aircraft. But you have a right to a good night's sleep and there are ways to minimize the problem.

It is sometimes difficult enough to wind down before going to sleep, without noise augmenting the problem. In crowded, bustling cities, background noise can make life a misery and lead to insomnia and bad dreams – but you can take steps to tackle the problem.

peace and quiet

If you live on a busy road, or under a flight path approach to a busy airport, choose the room furthest away from the road or air route to be your bedroom. It may be worth investing in double-glazing.

Terraced housing and poor flat conversions also present problems, as even the normal, everyday sounds of footsteps can echo irritatingly through adjoining flats or houses. To block out such sounds it is possible to install false walls or acoustic tiling – such as that used to soundproof recording studios – against party walls. This may seem an expensive and bothersome move, but in the long term, a consistent lack of sleep will always be more expensive in terms of energy and quality of life lost.

noisy neighbours

If your neighbours make a habit of playing loud music, or hammering and drilling late at night, the first step is to have a word with them and come to a reasonable compromise. Most people want to get on with their neighbours, and yours may have not realized that their activities were disturbing you.

For very raucous parties where gentle reminders have been ignored, it may be necessary to inform the

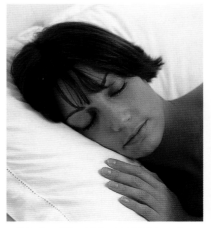

▲ Good-quality earplugs can help you to sleep undisturbed in a noisy environment.

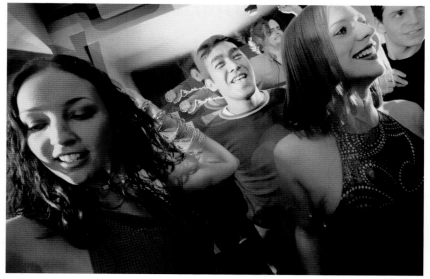

police, who will try to enforce some level of quiet. You may be able to ignore the occasional party, especially if you have been given a neighbourly warning, but regular late-night revelry does erode good will expecially if it affects your ability to get a decent night's sleep. As a general rule, it is customary to keep noise to a friendly minimum between the hours of 11pm and 8am. Some people need reminding of this, however. If the problem persists, you can take action through your local government.

earplugs

On those occasions when there is nothing you can do about the noise around you − if you are travelling and sleeping in a strange environment where the slightest sound keeps you awake − strange hotels for instance − a set of good-quality earplugs could be worth their weight in gold. It

▲ *Living in busy city or town centres, where young people congregate to socialize, can have a severe effect on sleep quality.*

probably isn't wise to rely on this solution too much at home, however, as they may prevent you from hearing noises that are designed to wake you up, such as a smoke alarm.

▼ *Noisy neighbours can wreak havoc on a quiet neighbourhood.*

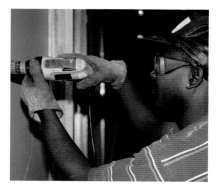

sedating aromas

Using an oil burner to disperse essential oils is a wonderfully fragrant way to calm an overactive mind and lull your tired body to sleep. Some essential oils have a gentle sedative effect.

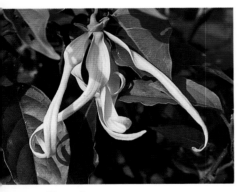

▲ *Ylang ylang.*

Oil burners come in many styles, but they all heat essential oil in water so that it vaporizes as steam and can be inhaled. Most contain a candle or nightlight, and they should never be left unattended or around an unsupervised child, and should not be left burning overnight.

blending oils
Relaxing, restorative oils to alleviate depression and nervous tension include basil, bergamot, camphor, chamomile, clary sage, jasmine, lavender, neroli, rose, sandalwood, thyme and ylang-ylang. Chamomile,

juniper, lavender, marjoram, neroli, rose and sandalwood have a sedative effect. Cedarwood, juniper, melissa, neroli, peppermint and rose are calming and uplifting.

You can use the oils on their own or in a combination of two or three to create a serene atmosphere. Place 6–8 drops of oil in the filled water chamber of the burner. Add more water and oil if necessary.

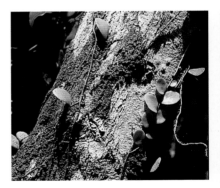

▲ *Camphor.*

STORAGE
Essential oils need to be kept in a cool place in airtight containers – dark glass bottles are best for long-term storage.

218 dispelling anger & anxiety

Negative feelings can leave you tossing and turning at night, instead of getting the rest you need. Aromatherapy oils can help dispel bad feelings before they cause sleepiness.

The ill effects of angry and anxious feelings can range from irritability and confusion, to impatience and explosive outbursts of rage. Coping with them is crucial for health.

dismantling anger

When allowed to fester, anger can certainly disturb sleep, so it is important to come to terms with the feeling and handle it in a positive, constructive way. Try to get to the root cause: why are you angry? Then think of ways to alleviate the feeling, i.e. expressing it calmly to another person. If you are angry with yourself over a mistake you may have made, remember that you are only human, and work on ways to rectify the situation that is troubling you.

diffusing anxiety

Stress and anxiety can be major factors in insomnia. Ongoing worries, perhaps over money or relationships, create tension that has a detrimental effect on your nervous system, outlook and sleeping patterns. If this anxious state continues, it can lead to illness.

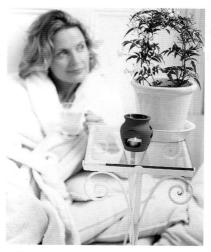

▲ Essential oils help to combat negativity and allow you to see things in perspective.

Regular exercise will help rid your system of the adrenalin produced by an anxious state, and meditation will help to restore your equilibrium. Relaxing essential oils – geranium, lavender and lemon – can help calm anger, while oils that are analgesic – basil, cedarwood, juniper and melissa – can help overcome fear and anxiety. Place a few drops in an oil burner or on a tissue and inhale the vapours.

To quell **feelings** of restlessness or irritation **at night,** place one or two drops of rose, **frankincense** or chamomile oil on to your **pillow.**

220 alleviating headaches & indigestion

Used in small amounts, pure essential oils can be added to hot tea to soothe away the stress of tension headaches and indigestion, thereby facilitating restful sleep.

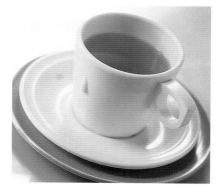

◄ If you find a cup of tea soothing, you can add to it the benefits of pure essential oils.

OIL TIPS
• Use only organic essential oils of therapeutic quality from a reputable source for adding to drinks.
• Absolutes or resins should never be ingested in this way.
• These methods should not be used for the treatment of children, but are suitable for the elderly.
• Never put essential oils directly into a drink, it will taste far too strong and will be very unpleasant.

To ease two common causes of restless sleep – headaches and stomach upset – pure essential oils can be added to a hot tea base. Choose oils that target the specific symptoms. For example, if you are suffering from indigestion, peppermint, fennel, chamomile and dill are all good choices. If your head is throbbing, lavender may ease the pain.

CAUTION
Do not increase the dosage without consulting a medical practitioner. The oils contain natural chemicals that are toxic in larger amounts.

making tea with oils
Tannin-free china or rooibos (red bush) tea make the best base for insomnia teas. Put 2–3 drops of essential oil on to the tea leaves or tea bag, add 1 litre/1¾ pints/4 cups of hot water, stir well, then remove the tea leaves or bag. The tea will taste best without milk.

Never pour essential oils directly into a cup of tea, as they will not disperse. Any tea that isn't drunk immediately may be stored in the refrigerator and reheated as required.

221 oils for insomnia

Not everyone needs an eight-hour quota of sleep, but if you find yourself awake night after night, perhaps due to a temporary problem or anxiety, aromatherapy oils may help.

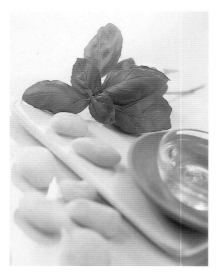

People have different sleep patterns, but if you do find yourself unable to sleep, whatever your natural pattern, the following essential oils can help, especially when added to a very warm bath at bedtime. Just add 4–6 drops to the water and swirl to disperse. Do not use the same oils for more than two weeks at a time.

▶ *Chamomile flowers have a gentle scent. Use the essential oil to help you sleep.*

◀ *Essential oils with sedative properties are an ideal addition to your evening bath.*

• **Basil:** This oil calms the nervous system generally.
• **Chamomile:** A very calming and relaxing oil, and a good choice when indigestion hinders sleep.
• **Clary sage:** This has a sedative and almost euphoric action, but do not use if you have had alcohol – it can give you nightmares or a hangover.
• **Lavender:** Not only very soothing, but also analgesic, so if you have any aches and pains that lead to insomnia, this oil is probably the best remedy.
• **Marjoram:** In large amounts it is quite sedating – but it can leave you feeling groggy, so use sparingly.

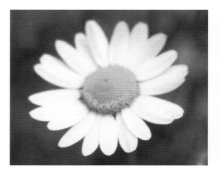

222 soothing massage oil

Aromatherapy essential oils can be combined with delicate carrier oils to help create a healing and comforting massage experience that can gently allow your body to wind down before bed.

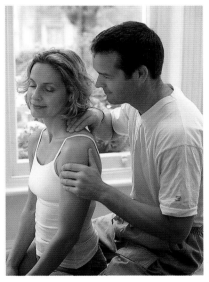

▲ The area around the neck and shoulders is particularly prone to holding tension.

A pleasant blend of lavender, clary sage and chamomile oils is ideal when you want to soothe away stress and help relieve feelings of nervous tension. Ideally, enjoy this oil as part of a full body massage, but when this is not possible, try gently massaging in a couple of drops of the oil behind the ears, using a circular motion.

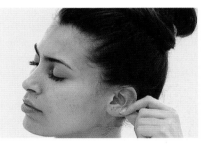

▲ Use a light carrier oil such as almond, and warm it gently in your hands before use.

tension–relieving massage oil
45ml/3 tbsp almond oil
1.5ml/¼ tsp wheatgerm oil
10 drops lavender, 5 drops clary sage,
    5 drops chamomile essential oil

Pour the almond and wheatgerm oils into a 50ml/2fl oz glass bottle, add the essential oils and gently shake to mix. Store in a cool, dark place.

> **CAUTION**
> Although generally safe, clary sage and chamomile oils should be avoided during pregnancy. If in doubt about any essential oils, consult a medical practitioner.

223 heavenly tubs

Being immersed in warm water is one of the most comforting sensations you can experience. For an antidote to a busy day, simply run a bedtime bath and enjoy the tranquillizing effects of water.

Many cultures throughout history have recognized the healing and health-giving properties of water, and spa resorts have been built around natural springs from ancient times to the present day. But you needn't be near a spa to enjoy water – a pampering and relaxing treat is only as far away as your own bathroom.

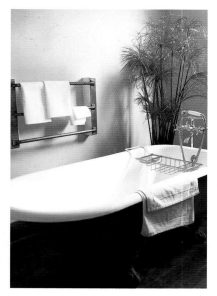

▲ Think of the bath as a place to relax and unwind as much as a place to get clean.

soothing waves

It is essential to find time to switch off from cares and worries. By reserving half an hour for yourself and locking the bathroom door, you can ensure a little oasis of peace while you read, listen to music or a play, or just lose yourself in pleasant contemplation – whatever you find most calming.

The ideal time for an evening bath is about an hour before going to sleep. This gives your body a chance to cool down slightly before you get into bed. Have big, fluffy towels on hand and a moisturizing cream or body oil to round off the sensual experience.

bathtime scenery

You can enhance your bathing pleasure by creating a room that cossets all your senses. Paint the room a watery colour, such as sea green or azure blue. If you like plants, surround the tub with moisture-loving ferns and scented plants such as jasmine or stephanotis. Soften lighting by fitting flattering amber, peach or pink lightbulbs, or use lanterns. Make sure the room is warm in winter, and well ventilated in summer.

224 sedative bath bags

Cloth bags filled with herb blossoms make a subtle and gentle addition to your evening bath – the sedative properties of these therapeutic plants wil help to soothe you to sleep.

A sleep-inducing mixture of lime, chamomile and hop flowers is a perfect wind down to an early night.

soporific bath bags
eight 30 x 10cm/12 x 4in rectangles
   of loosely woven fabric
needle and thread
50g/2oz chamomile flowers
50g/2oz lime blossom
25g/1oz hop flowers
50g/2oz coarse oatmeal
lengths of ribbon or string

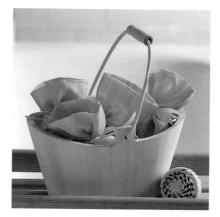

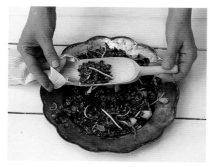

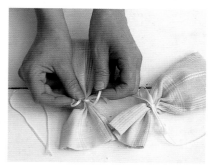

1 Fold the fabric rectangles in half and sew up three sides. Turn right-sides out. Combine the herbal ingredients and oatmeal and fill the bags with the mixture.

2 To finish, tie a large loop in a length of ribbon or string before using it to secure each bag. The loop can then be hung around the hot tap so that the running water flows through the bag. The materials make eight bags.

225 floral salts

A concoction of salts and aromatic flowers, herbs or oils can be added to the bath for a wonderful soak at bedtime. Although many salts are suitable, simple sea salt is used for this mixture.

Chamomile is a widely recognized sedative; for the following bath it has been combined with sweet marjoram, which is an effective treatment for insomnia.

These bath salts should be used only if you are planning to go straight to sleep after your bath: sweet marjoram is thought to be an anaphrodisiac, which means that it has the opposite effect of an aphrodisiac!

▼ As well as having a sedative effect, the bath salts will heal and stimulate the skin.

chamomile bath salts
500g/1¼lb/2½ cups coarse sea salt
10 drops chamomile essential oil
10 drops sweet marjoram essential oil
1–3 drops green or blue food
    colouring (optional)

Combine all the ingredients, mixing well with a wooden spoon, and pour into a glass jar with a lid. Place the lid on firmly and store in a cool place.

Add two heaped tablespoons of salts to the bath, pouring them under the hot tap as the water runs.

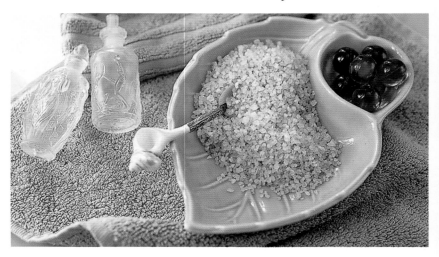

A few drops of lavender oil added to your bath will direct you towards slumber in a sumptuous cloud of scent.

227 easing herbal foot bath

Tired, sore feet can be a cause of wakefulness at night, especially if you have been standing or walking all day. A foot bath made with herbs is a soothing antidote that will help ease you to sleep.

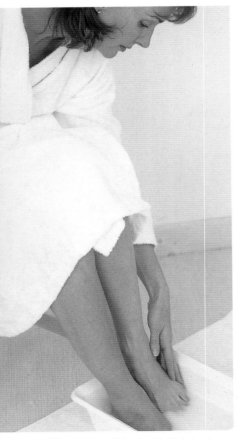

▲ A fragrant, soothing foot bath helps to warm and restore the whole body.

Peppermint is a particularly effective herb in foot baths. It has a cooling effect and helps to soothe aching muscles; rosemary is also useful for reducing pain. All the herbs listed will have a relaxing effect on the whole body as you inhale the fragrant steam rising from the hot water.

herbal foot bath for aching feet
50g/2oz mixed fresh herbs:
    peppermint, yarrow, pine needles,
    chamomile flowers, rosemary,
    houseleek
1 litre/1¾ pints/4 cups boiling water
15ml/1 tbsp borax
15ml/1 tbsp Epsom salts

Roughly chop all the fresh herbs, then place them in a bowl and pour the boiling water over them. Leave to stand for an hour. Strain the liquid, and add it to a bowl containing about 1.75 litres/3 pints/7½ cups hot water – the final temperature of the foot bath should be comfortably warm. Stir in the borax and the Epsom salts. Immerse the feet and soak them for about 15–20 minutes, then dry them thoroughly with a warm towel.

228 warming foot relaxer

A fragrant foot bath is ideal for refreshing tired feet. Not only does it comfort weary feet and calves, its warmth also relaxes the whole body and the scent of the herbs calms the mind.

The lavender in this mixture enhances feelings of serenity, and the lemon verbena restores balance to the nervous system.

lemon and lavender foot bath

15g/½oz dried lemon
    verbena leaves
30ml/2 tbsp dried lavender
30ml/2 tbsp cider vinegar
5 drops lavender essential oil

Place the lemon verbena and lavender in a basin and pour in enough hot water to cover the feet. When it has cooled to a comfortable temperature, add the cider vinegar and the lavender oil and swirl. Immerse the feet for 15–20 minutes, then dry well with a warm towel.

▾ *A comforting herbal foot bath can also help to alleviate the symptoms of a cold.*

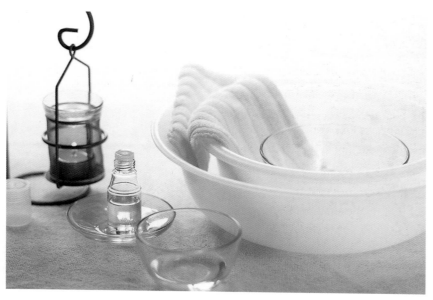

229 sleepy herbal pillow

A small pillow filled with calming herbs and flowers can help you to get to sleep at night. You will continue to benefit from its sedative effects all night, waking refreshed from untroubled sleep.

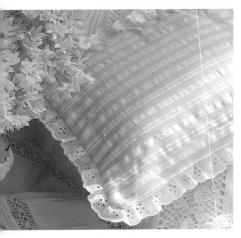

▲ Fill a small pillow with herbs so that you can benefit from their aroma as you sleep.

sleep potpourri

115g/4oz/2 cups dried hop flowers
115g/4oz/2 cups dried rose petals
50g/2oz/1 cup dried chamomile flowers
25g/1oz/½ cup each dried jasmine, orange blossom and lavender
10ml/2 tsp ground orris root
5ml/1 tsp frankincense powder
5–6 drops neroli essential oil

Mix the ingredients together. Place in an airtight container and leave in a warm, dry place for about ten days.

▼ Lavender is a useful sleep herb, lifting depression and alleviating stress.

Prepare the potpourri first. All the ingredients for this are available from health food suppliers and herbalists. When the scents have combined and the potpourri is ready, make up a muslin (cheesecloth) bag and loosely fill it with the mixture. You can slip this bag into your ordinary pillowcase, or stitch a special small pillow and slip the herbal bag inside it. Tuck the pillow under your neck to enjoy its aroma as you go to sleep.

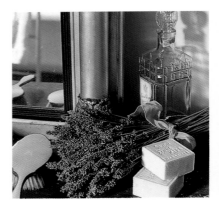

230 relaxing flower remedies

Bach flower remedies are vibrational essences. They work on the premise that natural energies can help redress emotional imbalances that may inhibit healthy functions such as sleep.

Developed by Dr Edward Bach in the early 20th century, Bach flower essences are sold individually or in mixtures designed to help alleviate specific complaints. The following remedies are prepared especially for sleep problems such as insomnia and nightmares. If you prefer, you can ask your health practitioner to create a tailor-made treatment for you.

fears and nightmares mix
This mixture is ideal for fears, night terrors and nightmares experienced by both adults and children. It contains a blend of Aspen, Cherry Plum, Mimulus, Rock Rose, Star of Bethlehem and White Chestnut.

insomnia mix
Used for releasing negative mental and emotional patterns, Insomnia mixture also works to soothe and quieten any excessive mental excitement that might prevent sleep. It contains Impatiens, Rock Rose, Vervain and White Chestnut.

morning glory
(*Ipomoea purpurea*)
This single flower essence can be useful if you are leading an erratic lifestyle. It works gently to support the body clock.

▾ The absorption of the flower's energy in water is activated by the action of sunlight.

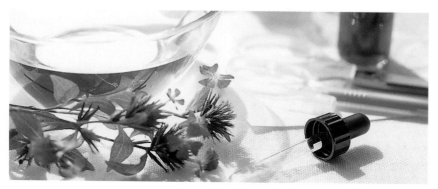

231 soothing lavender

The heady scent of lavender conjures up images of bountiful fields of blooms waving in the sunlight. But lavender has many uses: its healing and sedative qualities make it a key aid to natural sleep.

From ancient Egyptian times to the present day, lavender has been a star among medicinal plants. The Roman Pliny the Elder claimed that it was good for everything from dropsy to menstrual problems, and Elizabeth I drank lavender tea to cure migraines.

Lavender is still used in many herbal remedies. Cushions filled with dried lavender can help induce sleep,

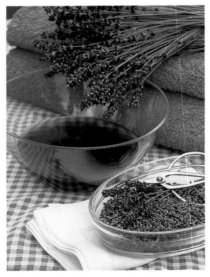

▲ An infusion of fresh or dried lavender flowers has relaxing qualities.

aid depression and alleviate stress; sniffing lavender oil sprinkled on a tissue has a similar effect. Fresh or dried flowers can be brewed into a tea that helps to cleanse the system and relieves headaches and stomach upsets. Lavender can also be made into a compress for external use to relieve sinus congestion, headaches, hangovers, tension and exhaustion.

If you are suffering from an evening headache or cold symptoms, or are feeling generally ill at ease, one of the following methods may help soothe you to sleep.

lavender infusion or tea
Pour boiling water into a cup, let it cool for 30 seconds, then add a teaspoonful of fresh or dried lavender. Cover the infusion and leave to steep for 10 minutes, stirring occasionally. Strain and drink the tea warm. Sweeten with a little honey if desired.

lavender compress
Soak a clean cloth in a hot infusion of lavender. Lie back and place the compress gently over your forehead, making sure not to get it in your eyes.

232 sleep-inducing violets

Tinctures are an effective way to extract the active medicinal constituents of plants. They keep well and may be taken when needed. This tincture uses sweet violets, which help to ease insomnia.

Tinctures are made by steeping the plant material in a mixture of water and alcohol. The alcohol draws out the active ingredients and also acts as a preservative. A 5ml/1 tsp dose of this remedy may be taken 3–4 times a day to relieve symptoms of insomnia and promote sound sleep.

sweet violet tincture
15g/½oz dried violet flowers
250ml/8fl oz/1 cup vodka
50ml/2fl oz/¼ cup water

1 Put the dried violet flowers into a glass jar, pour in the vodka and water then shake gently. The mixture will take on the a violet colour immediately.

2 Put a lid on the jar and leave in a cool, dark place for 7–10 days (no longer); shake occasionally. The tincture should darken.

3 Strain off the violets through a sieve lined with kitchen paper then pour the liquid into a sterilized glass bottle. Seal with a tight-fitting cork and store for future use in a cool, dark place. The tincture will keep for up to two years.

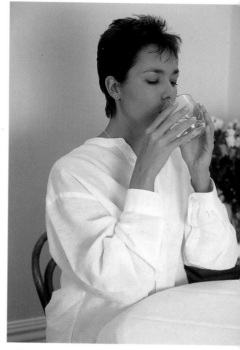

▲ You can add the tincture to a glass of water and sip slowly.

CAUTION
Never use industrial alcohol, or methylated or white spirits to make tinctures, as all these are highly toxic.

233 foods for restful sleep

You can help ensure sound sleep by eating from a variety of healthy foods throughout the course of the day. Avoiding foods that contain stimulants will also improve night-time rest.

bountiful sleep enhancers

Ensuring that your daytime diet is rich in B vitamins will help you sleep: the B group supports the nervous system and aids dream activity. Foods rich in Bs include green vegetables, nuts, seeds, eggs, seafood, soya, dairy foods and yeast extract.

Slow-burning carbohydrates such as oats, barley, rice and beans provide the body with a steady release of energy that helps keep the system on an even keel all day.

regulating the sleep cycle

Tryptophan is an amino acid found in turkey, milk, tuna fish and most carbohydrates. If there are sufficient levels of vitamin B6 in the body, tryptophan will aid in the production of neurotransmitters such as serotonin, which helps to regulates sleep patterns.

Calcium also helps release such serotonin. Choose foods such as broccoli, oats, sesame seeds, tahini and raw vegetables, rather than dairy products, which tend to increase mucus production. Kelp and other seaweeds are a rich source of calcium, as are watercress, dandelions and nettle.

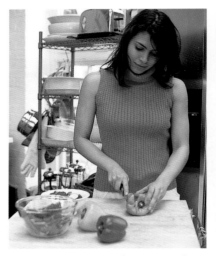

▲ Eat raw vegetables and unprocessed food throughout the day.

OVERSTIMULATING FOODS
It is best to avoid these substances
• **Caffeine:** this potent drug can make you edgy and irritable; avoid after 2–4pm.
• **Sugar:** refined sugars disturb metabolic processes; substitute honey, fruit sugars or maple syrup.
• **Chemical additives:** these are difficult for your body to process and may keep you awake.

234 perfect night-time food

Alhough doctors maintain that eating a large meal late at night is harmful to the system, hunger pangs can be a cause of wakefulness. A light snack provides the perfect solution.

When restlessness is due to a rumbling stomach, the best remedy is to treat yourself to a midnight snack. Stick to light foods – try wholemeal (wholewheat) crackers spread with a little peanut butter and a hot, milky drink. A small sandwich filled with turkey, avocado or cottage cheese is ideal, as these contain tryptophan, which may assist healthy sleep. Other easy-to-digest foods include a bowl of comforting oatmeal or a banana.

It is best to avoid foods that are difficult to digest, such as meats and high-fat content cheeses, or rich foods such as heavy sauces, pastries and cakes. Very sugary or acidic foods may give you heartburn, which will keep you awake. Always sit up for 15–20 minutes after eating before going back to bed, to give the food a chance to travel down the intestines.

drink up

Caffeine is best avoided from mid-afternoon onwards, but in general, hot drinks have a calming effect at bedtime, especially in cold weather. If you wake frequently in the night, a flask filled with a hot, caffeine-free

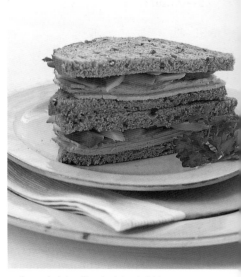

▲ A sandwich will calm late night hunger pangs, but pick an easily digestible filling.

drink such as herbal tea, chicory "coffee" or plain hot water can provide an instant soother. It also means that you needn't get up, thus making it easier to return to sleep.

If your wakefulness is due to sultry weather, iced chamomile or lemon balm tea will cool you down and provide instant relief.

237 soothing tisanes

Made by steeping garden-fresh flowers in boiling water, tisanes provide a real treat for the taste buds. They can calm the nerves and send you to sleep on a proverbial carpet of blossoms.

The experience of drinking a tisane is a little like taking the garden's earthy energy into your system. The wonderful fragrances of these clean and clear tonics act as mood enhancers, and they are visually cheering – as well as tasting wonderfully fresh. Many garden blossoms can be used for making tisanes, but the best ones for promoting sound sleep include: lavender, lime blossom, lemon verbena, dandelion, rosemary, rose petals, jasmine, peppermint, bergamot and passion flower.

> Flower teas can be made from dried flowers when fresh blooms are not in season.

passion flower tisane

The passion flower has wonderful sedative powers that are said to relieve nervous conditions such as palpitations and shakiness, thus helping to prevent insomnia.

To make a tisane, place one passion flower blossom (or 5ml/1 tsp dried passion flower) in a cup and add 250ml/8 fl oz/1 cup boiling water. Steep for 10 minutes, then remove the flower. You can drink a cup of this soothing tisane 3 times a day, and continue for 2–4 weeks.

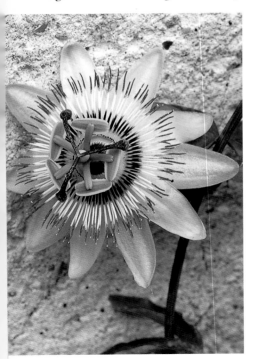

◀ For the best tisanes, cut passion flowers when the plant is producing its fruit.

238 warming eggnog

This Scandinavian/American drink is usually served cold, but this is a warm and creamy version, guaranteed to soothe and relax on a chilly autumn or winter's night.

Delicious eggnog is spicy and rich, so a little goes a long way – a normal serving is about the size of a small wineglass. Drunk in the evening after dinner, it provides an ideal way to wind down before bedtime. The drink can also be made without alcohol – substitute 7.5ml/1½ tsp of rum flavouring for the rum.

warming eggnog

serves 2

250ml/8fl oz/1 cup double (heavy) cream
1 long strip orange rind
1.5ml/¼ tsp freshly grated nutmeg
1 cinnamon stick
2 eggs, separated
30ml/2 tbsp caster (superfine) sugar
75ml/2½fl oz/⅓ cup golden rum
cinnamon sticks to serve

Warm the glasses. Pour the cream into a small pan; add the orange rind, nutmeg and cinnamon stick and bring slowly to the boil. In a mixing bowl, beat the egg yolks with the sugar until really pale and creamy. When the cream is boiling, pour on to the egg mixture and whisk well.

Return the mixture to the pan and stir over a very gentle heat until it forms a custard as thick as pouring cream. Do not overheat the mixture or it will curdle. Warm the rum in another pan. Stir it into the egg custard, then whisk the egg whites until soft peaks form, and fold them into the hot custard. Serve in the warm glasses, with a cinnamon stick.

▼ *Thick creamy eggnog, laced with rum, is a delicious nightcap for a cold evening.*

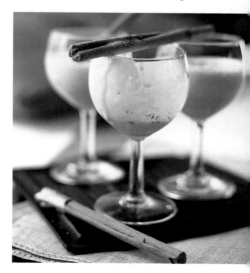

239 comforting hot drinks

When indulged in occasionally, a hot, alcoholic beverage can go a long way towards directing you to restful sleep. It is especially good when you are suffering from a cold.

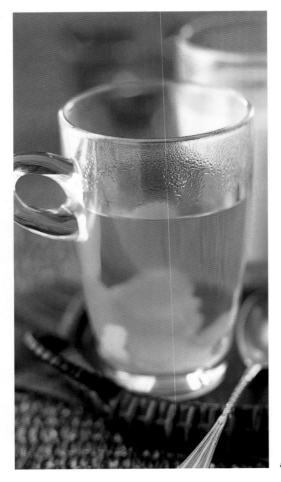

hot toddy

serves 2

2 strips lemon rind
4 slices fresh root ginger
5ml/1 tsp honey
175ml/6fl oz/¾ cup water
175ml/6fl oz/¾ cup
   whiskey or bourbon

Put the lemon rind, ginger, honey and water in a small pan and bring to the boil. Remove the pan and leave for 5 minutes. Stir in the alcohol and allow time for it to warm through. Rest a silver spoon in each pre-heated glass and strain in the warm toddy. Sip slowly.

CAUTION
As with all alcoholic beverages the sedative effect will be reversed if you consume too much alcohol.

◄ *A hot toddy will warm you up and relax tired muscles.*

240 sweet nutmeg milk

Milk contains substances that help restore feelings of calmness. When drunk at bedtime it can enhance restful sleep. The additions of honey and nutmeg give a soothing and tasty twist.

The first food that we consume as babies, milk has a soothing effect on the nervous system. It contains peptides that help to relieve stress and anxiety, and reduce nervous tension that can lead to insomnia. Many people find milk helpful in cases of indigestion – another common cause of wakefulness – particularly if it is sipped warm.

When drunk with honey and a sprinkling of nutmeg, a mug of warm milk makes a perfect bedtime nightcap. If you suffer from an allergy or sensitivity to dairy products, you can substitute goat, soya or oat milk for cow's milk.

hot nutmeg milk
This recipe makes one serving, but you can easily multiply the ingredients for two or more people. Heat 250ml/8fl oz/1 cup whole or semi-skimmed (low fat) milk in a milk pan, to just below the boiling point – do not scald. Remove from the heat and whisk until frothy. Stir in 10ml/2 tsp clear honey, then pour into a large mug and grate a light dusting of nutmeg over the milk.

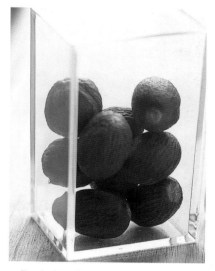

▲ For the best flavour, always buy whole nutmeg and grate it as you need it.

> **CAUTION**
> Use nutmeg sparingly. Although in small amounts its active ingredient, myristicin, enhances sleep and pleasant dreams, in large doses it is highly toxic. Just one to three grated nutmegs (in excess of 5ml/1tsp) can cause hallucinations, nausea and vomiting.

241 sleep pattern crystal cure

Sleeplessness can be brought on by a variety of causes. With the help of healing crystals, the situation can be overcome and your sleep patterns brought into balance once more.

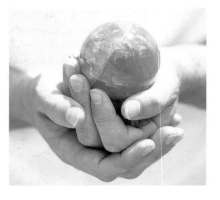

Different gemstones are said to ease various physical ailments, including disturbances in sleep patterns. The best way to use crystals is to get to know them by experimenting with them individually – one that works well for you may keep someone else awake. When you are half asleep and exhausted, the motivation to help yourself can be difficult to summon up. Having the right crystals at your bedside may help, so that you can simply pick one up without having to get out of bed.

▶ *Healing and calming, apple green chrysoprase encourages deep sleep.*

◀ *Holding an appropriate gemstone can help you relax and fall asleep.*

peaceful slumber

Chrysoprase has been found to encourage peaceful sleep. A tumbled stone can be put under your pillow, or on your bedside table.

When you are fearful, use a grounding and protecting stone such as tourmaline, staurolite, smoky quartz or tourmaline quartz and place it at the foot of your bed.

If tension and worry are causes of restlessness, amethyst, rose quartz or citrine may help. If your sleep pattern has been broken or disturbed by something you have eaten, a digestive calmer such as ametrine, moonstone or iron pyrites may be the solution.

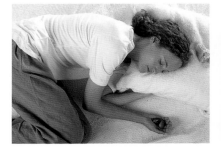

242 heart-healing crystals

There are many times in life when you may feel unhappy or heartsick, unable to do or say what you wish to. Healing crystals may help soothe the emotions so that you can sleep.

This layout of crystals is said to help calm an emotional upset and allow you to focus on a practical solution. As you work through it, you may notice signs of stress being relieved, including fluttering eyelids, deep sighs, twitching muscles, or yawning. Do not be alarmed if tearfulness results as aching feelings are released.

calming the heart
To clear emotional stress, you will need four clear quartz stones, a citrine, a small rose quartz and an amethyst. On the centre of the chest, place the rose quartz and surround it with four clear quartz points. If the points are placed facing outwards, they remove emotional imbalances. If they face inwards, they stabilize an over-emotional state. Just below the navel, place the citrine quartz with its point directed downwards, to increase a sense of security. Place the amethyst on the brow or above the top of the head to help calm the mind. If the release is too strong, remove the stones from the heart area and place a hand over the solar plexus.

▾ Use this powerful crystal layout to help you cope when you are feeling unhappy.

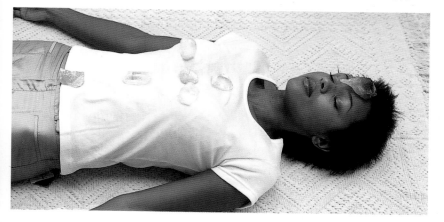

243 balancing & calming stones

After a hard day at work or with children, it can be difficult to wind down and relax. A simple placement of stones may help you to feel calm and refreshed after only a few minutes.

balancing the system

The three crystals used in this layout are all powerful healing stones and are useful in many situations. Clear quartz is said to quieten the mind and increase clarity, allowing you to

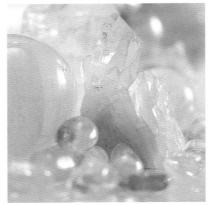

▲ Quartz is one of the most common healing stones available.

neutralize the day's negative events, and put both positive and negative into perspective. Used pointing downwards, smoky quartz helps to release tension and re-establishes focus on the present, allowing you to take greater enjoyment in your leisure time. Rose quartz is said to balance the chakra system and the emotions, and is good for removing blocked emotional stress.

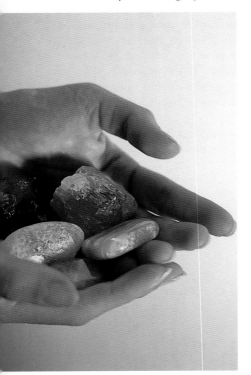

◀ Clean stones in fresh running water first.

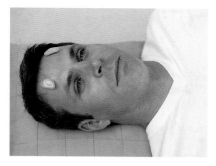

Place a clear quartz crystal, with its point upwards, above the top of the head. Place a smoky quartz crystal, point downwards, close to the base of the spine (between the upper thighs or knees), then place a small rose quartz crystal on the centre of the chest. After 4–5 minutes, you should find that you feel refreshed and in tune with yourself again.

◀ Just a few minutes spent each day focusing on relaxing will help calm you down.

stress release points

For the rapid, safe release of particular stresses, lie down in a peaceful spot. Place small rose quartz stones on the slightly raised bumps to the sides of the forehead. You may need to tape the stones in place. Take a deep breath to calm yourself. Remembering the stressful event will begin the release process, which will be complete when you feel a change of emotion or a return of equilibrium. Placing a grounding stone by the feet and a balancing stone at the heart, or solar plexus chakra, may also help.

▼ Clusters of amethyst are good to place in rooms as a focus for peace.

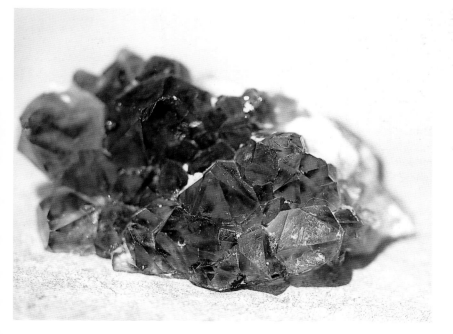

244 dealing with bad dreams

There are phases in everyone's life when they may be subject to bad dreams and nightmares. It is helpful to try to take a cool look at what these dreams might mean in the light of day.

Nightmares and fretful dreams often occur when life is in a state of upheaval. They may be due to anxiety about a current arrangement or the outcome of an upcoming event, or unresolved feelings or worries about yourself or other people.

The death of a loved one, illness, the end of a relationship, moving house, changing jobs, having a baby or getting married can all dredge up fears and anxieties. Even if a change is positive, it may produce anxious dreams that relay fears about your ability to "move with the times".

hidden obstacles

Sometimes bad dreams indicate the unconscious mind's attempt to bring hidden fears to the conscious mind, where they can be dealt with. In cases of long-term stress, bad dreams can bring the unresolved issues causing the problem to the surface. If you can make sense of your dream, you can try to apply what you've learned to your waking life.

Dreams can be an early warning system – they let you know when you need to reassess and de-stress. If

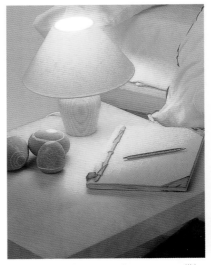

▲ If you write down your dreams, you will be able to ponder their meaning the next day.

you wake frightened or unnerved after a bad dream, turn on the light and assure yourself that you are awake and unharmed. It can be helpful to jot down the dream, thus "removing" it from your mind and on to the paper. If you have continual nightmares over a long period, you may wish to seek help from a therapist or counsellor to explore the underlying causes.

common scenarios

When feelings prey on our minds, they are often reflected in dreams, which are mildly disturbing: taking a test; discovering a loved one in the arms of another; being inappropriately dressed at a social gathering, or ignored at a party; running but not moving. More dramatic nightmares include being chased by something or somebody; trying and failing to get somewhere; exams, tests or interviews that go horribly wrong, or for which you are unprepared; experiencing or witnessing violence; being strangled or suffocated; feeling paralysed or unable to move or escape.

physiological triggers

Bad dreams are sometimes triggered by physiological factors. Eating rich food before going to bed can lead to indigestion and disturb the quality of our sleep; heavy drinkers who give up alcohol may suffer frightening dreams for a while afterwards; and certain drugs, such as beta-blockers, can increase the frequency of bad dreams.

personality factors

Some people go through their lives having very few nightmares. So why is it that some of us suffer from them more than others? Dream studies have suggested that those who are more prone to nightmares are "thin-skinned". They are sensitive, apprehensive people who suffer a high level of tension in their waking lives. There also appears to be a link between types of personalities and types of nightmares. For example, high achievers are said to have more fantastic, dramatic nightmares. Women have also been found to be more prone to nightmares than men. It is perhaps not surprising that feelings of hopelessness, or of being threatened, are more common in women's dreams than in men's.

▾ *Left and below: Dreams have important messages for us. Keep paper and a pencil at the side of your bed. Write down the events and your feelings about those events, when they wake you. Analyze your dream later, keeping your current situation in mind.*

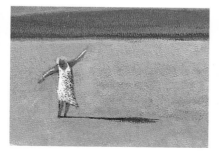

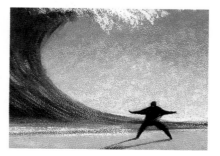

245 dream journal

Recording your dreams can give you valuable insights into the fabric of your dream life, tracing patterns that occur over time. It can also bring unconscious thoughts and needs into focus.

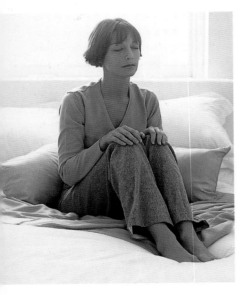

◄ *Work with your dream during the day, to try and bring it into focus and under control.*

to recall and replay it in a relaxed and conscious state, as being at ease makes your intuition flow more freely. Try sitting or lounging on the bed. Quiz the characters and places of the dream for answers to your questions: "Who are you? Why are you here? What are you trying to tell me?" Go with the first answers that pop into your mind, and try to apply them to your current situation; the dream's meaning should start to come into focus. Sometimes it takes a week or two of looking at a dream for its meaning to be digested and understood. The many books available on dream analysis and interpretation may help you explore dream symbolism further.

Write down your dreams as soon as you wake, whether in the middle of the night, or first thing in the morning. Dreams have a very elusive quality and tend to slip away almost immediately, so it is best to capture them as soon as possible.

exploring the unknown

Use your journal to work with a dream when you are awake. You need

creative voice

Remember, dreams can be a vehicle for synthesizing ideas – people have been known to write great stories, compose beautiful music and solve scientific puzzles via their dreams, so recording them may lend inspiration for your future endeavours.

246 calling an angel protector

It can be very comforting to visualize a protective spirit or "guardian angel" before going to sleep. This could be any figure you feel will watch over you and keep you safe during the night.

Especially when you are feeling vulnerable, lonely, ill or troubled, it can be helpful to visualize the presence of someone who protects you as you sleep. This protector could be a traditional angel figure, or it could be a missed loved one such as a parent or grandparent. It could even be a strong animal – perhaps a bear or a cougar.

The following exercise will help you create a force field of light that surrounds you in your mind's eye, with your angel or protector nearby.

angelic light
While in bed, relax completely, lying flat on your back. Rest your arms at your sides and take a few deep breaths. Imagine a strong and powerful figure, one for whom you feel complete trust and friendship. Visualize your protector's features; talk to them, and feel their calming presence reassure you. You may want to point out anything that is particularly bothering you, and know

that your protector understands and wants what is best for you.

Now imagine your body surrounded by a pool of bluish-white light. The light envelopes you completely with its beauty and serenity. Let the light spread out to surround your bed, in pulsating waves of energy. Know that the protector watches over you and the light, guarding your sleeping self and keeping you from harm.

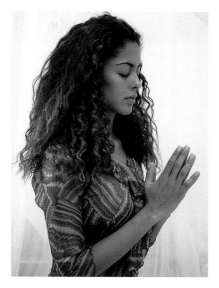

▸ *Call on your guardian angel before you go to bed to watch over you as you sleep.*

247 sleep cures

When slumber eludes you and you are left tossing and turning, it's time to rethink your bedtime tactics. Try adding one or more new practices to help you achieve a healthy night's sleep.

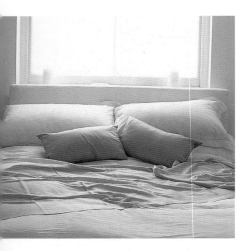

◀ *Try keeping your bed as a place for sleep only and rid the room of any distractions.*

can see fish swimming past.
• Visualize a boring scenario, such as a lecture you have no interest in.
• Read out loud the names and numbers from the phone book.
• Reserve your bedroom and the bed as a place for sleep only.
• Wiggle your toes gently until you fall asleep.
• Rub your stomach lightly.
• Cut up a mild onion, place in a jar by the bed and sniff before retiring.
• Think of ten wonderful things that have happened to you today.
• Squeeze all your muscles together tightly for a few minutes then relax.

instant fixes

If all else fails and you are still awake in the dead of night, try some, or all, of these quick cures.
• Lie on your back with your knees propped on a small pillow.
• Sleep with your head facing north.
• Get up at the same time every morning and go to bed at the same time every night for a week.
• Visualize yourself in a peaceful place, such as a field full of wildflowers with a gentle breeze blowing, or near a gently flowing stream where you

CAUTION

Avoid these sleep deterrents:
• Drinking excessive alcohol
• Smoking cigarettes
• Taking long naps in the afternoon
• Watching disturbing films or TV prior to bed
• Playing video games
• Listening to fast-paced or loud music

248 prayer for sleep

By reaching out to your god or the universe with a prayer before sleep, you will experience feelings of peaceful release and freedom from worry. Chanting can also help to set your mind at rest.

Many faiths have formal bedtime prayers – such as the Christian "Now I lay me down to sleep" – that are designed to comfort the individual and lend a feeling of protection during the seven or eight hours' absence from consciousness. This is a nice way to round off the day and complete your thoughts.

protection prayer
I ask God, the stars in the sky and the
    moon above
to look down upon me and all I love
to watch and protect us throughout
    the night
to keep us from danger and
fill our hearts and souls with golden
    light.

bedtime chant
Let me move beyond cares
Let me leave fear behind
Let me rest in a peaceful land
Let me wander to the farthest shores
    of dreams, to learn what I will and
    see what I see
then safely return when morning
    comes,
refreshed and ready for a new dawn.

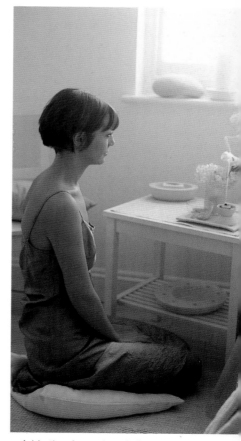
▲ Add a time for contemplation or prayer to your bedtime ritual.

249 lull yourself to sleep

At the end of a hectic day, soothing music can help you wind down in a pleasant way. Likewise, a blanket of neutral sound can help drown out the rest of the world, allowing deep relaxation.

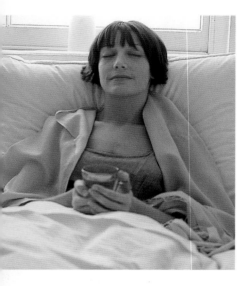

◄ *Listen to your relaxing sounds as you sip a cup of herbal tea, or after you settle down.*

Listening to pieces of classical music before bed may help you drift off to sleep. Music played on a single instrument, such as *Slow Pieces for Spanish Guitar* by Fernando Sor or piano pieces by Claude Debussy or Eric Satie, are good choices. New Age music is also ideal – often slow and repetitive, it brings a meditative state.

Make a tape or CD containing your favourite pieces of music. Avoid anything with a fast beat or sudden tempo changes. The more similar the pieces are in tempo and "feel", the more soporific will be the effect, as the repetition of similar notes will make your mind de-focus.

natural music
The sounds found in nature can have a hypnotic effect – very beneficial just before you go to bed. CDs are available containing sounds, such as the jungle, bird calls and whale songs. The sounds of the seashore are particularly relaxing and evocative.

calming noise
Some people find that white noise helps to curb the effects of environmental noise, such as background traffic or inconsiderate neighbours. Tune a radio to between stations, to where you will hear a hiss and turn the volume low. Alternatively, leave a fan running – its hum has a similar effect. If you find it comforting to hear people, leave on a talk radio station at a very low volume.

If you have a persistent **dream** try challenging it during the day. Light a **candle** to help you **focus** your thoughts, and consciously **relive** the dream. When you reach the disturbing part, take **control** and change the ending to a **happier** one.

index

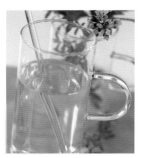

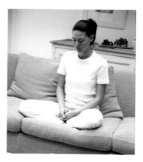

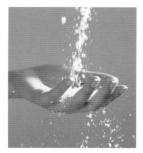

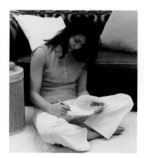

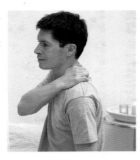